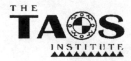

Introduction To
Taos Institute Publications

The Taos Institute is a nonprofit organization dedicated to the development of social constructionist theory and practices for purposes of world benefit. Constructionist theory and practice locate the source of meaning, value, and action in communicative relations among people. Chief importance is placed on relational process and its outcomes for the welfare of all. Taos Institute Publications offers contributions to cutting-edge theory and practice in social construction. These books are designed for scholars, practitioners, students, and the openly curious. The **Focus Book Series** provides brief introductions and overviews that illuminate theories, concepts, and useful practices. The **Books for Professionals Series** provides in-depth works, which focus on recent developments in theory and practice. Books in both series are particularly relevant to social scientists and to practitioners concerned with individual, family, organizational, community, and societal change.

Kenneth J. Gergen
President, Board of Directors
The Taos Institute

For information about the Taos Institute visit: www.taosinstitute.net

Taos Institute Publications

Focus Book Series

The Appreciative Organization, (2001) by Harlene Anderson, David Cooperrider, Kenneth J. Gergen, Mary Gergen, Sheila McNamee, and Diana Whitney

Appreciative Leaders: In the Eye of the Beholder, (2001) Edited by Marge Schiller, Bea Mah Holland, and Deanna Riley

Experience AI: A Practitioner's Guide to Integrating Appreciative Inquiry and Experiential Learning, (2001) by Miriam Ricketts and Jim Willis

Appreciative Sharing of Knowledge: Leveraging Knowledge Management for Strategic Change, (2004) by Tojo Thatchekery

Social Construction: Entering the Dialogue, (2004) by Kenneth J. Gergen and Mary Gergen

Dynamic Relationships: Unleashing the Power of Appreciative Inquiry in Daily Living, (2005) by Jacqueline M. Stavros and Cheri B. Torres

Appreciative Inquiry: A Positive Approach to Building Cooperative Capacity, (2005) by Frank J. Barrett, Ph.D. and Ronald E. Fry

Books for Professionals Series

SocioDynamic Counselling: A Practical Guide to Meaning Making, (2004) by R. Vance Peavy

Experiential Exercises in Social Construction – A Fieldbook for Creating Change, (2004) by Robert Cottor, Alan Asher, Judith Levin, and Cindy Weiser

Dialogues About a New Psychology, (2004) by Jan Smedslund

Therapeutic Realities: Social Construction and the Therapeutic Process, (2006) by Kenneth J. Gergen

For on-line ordering of books from Taos Institute Publications visit www.taospub.net or www.taosinstitute.net/publishing/publishing.html

For further information, write or call:
1-888-999-TAOS, 1-440-338-6733, info@taosinstitute.net or taosinstitutepublishing@alltel.net

Therapeutic Realities

Collaboration, Oppression
And Relational Flow

Kenneth J. Gergen

Taos Institute Publications

Chagrin Falls, Ohio

USA

THERAPEUTIC REALITIES:
Collaboration, Oppression And Relational Flow

COVER ART: Designed by Anne Marie Rijsman-Lecluse
and reproduced with permission

Copyright © 2006 Kenneth J. Gergen

The major contents of this book were first published in 2005 in the French language as, Construrire la Realite, Un nouvel avenir pour la psychotherapie. All non-English rights are the possession of the publisher, Editions du Seuil.

Taos Institute Publications
Chagrin Falls, Ohio

ISBN: 0-7880-2166-4
LCN: 2005934529

PRINTED IN U.S.A.

Table Of Contents

Preface

The present volume grows out of more than three decades of dialogue with therapists from around the world. I have entered these dialogues as a scholar with a deep concern for the consequences of intellectual work for societal practices. It has been most gratifying to me that therapists have found my inquiries into social construction valuable in deliberating about their efforts. More importantly, because they have invited me into their dialogues, my understanding has increased manifold and the ideas both sharpened and enriched. I must say as well, that my appreciation for the challenge of therapeutic work has similarly increased. My work as a scholar seems far easier by comparison. I arrange words on the page and return the next day to find them just as I left them. Each day I can re-shape, and never is there decomposition in my absence. In contrast, the therapist works with an ever-shifting subject; change may be mercurial and multiplicative. I deeply admire therapeutic accomplishments.

My scholarly work has chiefly been dedicated to exploring the relational origins of meaning, how it is that we come to understand the world and ourselves in the way we do, why such understandings are so often intractable, and how it is possible to bring about change. Such work not only bears on the philosophical problem of knowledge, along with the political problem of individualism. It is also central to anyone concerned with personal or social change. As a philosophic inquiry, my work joins hands with significant developments in both the sociology of knowledge and the history of science that question the longstanding assumptions of objectivity, rationality, and empirical truth. If our accounts of the world are generated within human relationships, then these accounts are not so much mirrors or pictures of the world, but means by which human beings appropriate the world for their purposes. In this respect, claims to objectivity, rationality and truth can be established and legitimated only within communities. For those standing outside such communities, such claims may not only be misguided but actively oppressive.

As a political endeavor my work is first set against the longstanding tradition of Western individualism. If all meaning is brought forth within relational process, as I propose, then the very concept of an individual mind is essentially derivative of relationship. Politically this line of argument not only lends itself to contemporary critiques of individualist ideology, but invites as well the development of alternative realities. More pointedly, our attention is directed to the significance of relationship in giving birth to the individual, sustaining our ways of life, and as a fulcrum to personal change.

Moving from issues of politics and ideology to practices of therapy, my thinking has benefited especially from major moves in the therapeutic world. The first of these is the constructivist movement, inspired initially by George Kelly, but enriched and expanded significantly through the works of Umberto Maturana, Ernst von Glasersfeld, Michael Mahoney, Robert Neimeyer, and many others. In challenging the realist assumptions so central to the therapeutic tradition, constructivist writings opened the door to considering multiple constructions of the world. While the individualist roots of constructivism contrast sharply with the social constructionist ideas so central to my writings, a rich and gratifying dialogue has ensued.

The second important development in the therapeutic world was in its shift from an individual to a systemic understanding of human problems. This movement, from the early writings of Gregory Bateson, through the work of the Milan School, and both first and second order cybernetics, illuminated the possibilities of a relational orientation to therapy. Again, such work also opened the door to dialogues with social construction, and the attempt to move beyond individualist ontology. In this case, constructionist ideas invited a shift in systemic thinking toward the relational genesis of meaning and the pivotal place of language within this process.

The constructionist concern with language also lent itself to a third domain of dialogue, namely with therapists who had become engaged with various strands of postmodern, post-foundational and post-structural thought. In many respects, my constructionist ideas have come to fruition in precisely this milieu. Thus, I was invited into highly congenial dialogues with narrative therapists, brief therapists, postmodern therapists and others of related persuasion. It is the fruits of these three lines of dialogue—with constructivists, systemicists, and the discursively oriented—that will largely be shared within the present volume.

The chapters in this work are largely based on contributions I have made to various books and journals over the past decade. In each case, however, I have reworked the material, elaborating and editing so as to reflect current deliberations, and orchestrating the chapters to form a coherent whole. In Part I of the volume I include attempts at understanding therapeutic process and practice from a social constructionist perspective. The initial chapter, on therapeutic communication, was written especially for this book. It first introduces several major components of social constructionist thought, and then provides what, for most readers, will be a novel account of therapeutic communication. This account is an important cornerstone of the book, in that it enables us to move beyond traditional conceptions of inter-subjectivity to a radical relationalism.

The second chapter grows from the soil of an earlier book, Therapy as Social Construction (Sage, 1992), edited with Sheila McNamee. This volume, now appearing in six languages, made initial inroads into linking constructionist thought with specific therapeutic practices. It was this book that led to my joining Lisa Warhus, a clinical psychologist then residing in Denmark, to carry out a full-scale analysis of emerging therapeutic practices from a constructionist standpoint. Our work was subsequently published in Sistemas Familiares in 2001. The present chapter is an updating and reworking of that material.

As noted above, there is a strong affinity between constructionist ideas and the narrative movement in therapy. Chapter 3 explores this connection in some detail. Importantly, however, the attempt here is to press beyond current understanding of the significance of narrative. The initial drafting of this material was enriched greatly by John Kaye, a therapist/ scholar from Adelaide, Australia, and was published in my earlier book, Realities and Relationships (Harvard University Press, 1994)

In Part II I include two chapters that treat what I see as enormously oppressive and injurious aspects of the current mental health establishment. Chapter 4, on deficit discourse, furnishes a critical analysis of the diagnostic movement in mental health. From a constructionist standpoint, the consequences of psychodiagnostic categorization are deeply injurious to the culture, offering myriad means by which common problems are reconstituted as mental illness. Again, an earlier draft of this work appeared in Realities and Relationships. Chapter 5 continues in this critical vein by considering more recent moves to define mental illness in terms of neurological deficits. Here I try to illuminate the illusory character of such reductionism, and to trace the inimical effects of the neuro/ biological construction on human society. This chapter was written especially for this volume.

In Part III of the book, I include four chapters treating more specialized topics in relational process. Chapter 6 explores the poetic dimension of therapeutic communication. Here it is argued that by viewing language as poetry, we gain insight into the use of language in bringing about change. An earlier version of this chapter appeared in a volume edited by Klaus Deissler and Sheila McNamee, Phil und Sopie auf der Couch. Die sociale Poesie therapeutischer Gesprache (Carl-Auer, 2000). Chapter 7, on reflexive cooperation, is the result of a recent collaboration with Eugene Epstein, a friend and colleague since our meeting in Heidelberg some 15 years ago. The case material Eugene provides, places much needed flesh on the theoretical bones of social construction. An earlier draft of this paper appears in German, in Familien-dynamik (2005).

In the final chapters of the volume, I include interview discussions with two internationally prominent therapists, therapists for whom I have the deepest respect. The first discussion is with Mony Elkaim, a leader in the development of family therapy in Europe. The interview addresses important issues in constructionist applications to therapy, and makes useful links to significant lines of European thought. An earlier draft of the interview appeared in <u>Resonances</u>. April, 1996. In the final chapter, Michael Hoyt, a prominent figure in the development of constructive therapies, addresses a range of specific issues in constructionist thought and application. This chapter is also important because it opens discussion on metaphysical implications of a constructionist orientation. The chapter is an excerpt from Hoyt's interview in <u>Interviews with brief therapy experts</u>. (Brunner-Routledge, 2001).

For whatever insight and wisdom one may find within these pages I am indebted to countless therapist/scholars with whom I have been engaged over the past 30 years. I have been graced by the insights of Sheila McNamee, John Kaye, Lynn Hoffman, Lisa Warhus, Eugene Epstein, and Roberta Iversen, all of whom have joined with me in various publishing efforts. At the same time, my understanding of the therapeutic process has been enriched manifold from conversations over the years with countless colleagues and friends within the profession. I shall certainly not recall all these at one sitting, but the following are memorable and significant:

Corin Ahlers , Tom Andersen , Saliha Bava, Lucien Barrolet. Lenore Behar, Elsa Bennested, Espen Bennested, Tom Cottle, Philip Cushman, Gianfranco Ceccin, Klaus Deissler, Lothar Dudah, Mony Elkaim, Eugene Epstein, Edna Foa, Saul Fuks. Jane Flax, Mary Fox, Norman Garmezey, Anne Gergen, Patrice Gherovici, Miguel Goncalves, James Griffith, Melissa Griffith, Jay Haley, Lois Holzman, Alan Holmgren, Marie Hoskins, Michael Hoyt, Bettina Iversen, Arlene Katz, Gerda Klammer, Joel Kovel, Peter Lang, Susan Levin, Michael Mahoney, Stan Messer,

Donald Meichenbaum, Steve Mitchell, Mary Blanca Moctezuma, Robert Neimeyer, Fred Newman, Bill O'Hanlon, Marcelo Pakman, David Paré, Vance Peavy, Peggy Penn, Stuart Pizer, Christina Ravazolla, Eero Riikonen, Alain Robiolio, Eliot Rodnick, Karin Roth, Sallyann Roth, Louis Sass, Karl Scheibe, Dora Schnitman, Jaco Seikulla, Ilene Serlin, Carlos Sluzki, Jan Smedslund, Michael Smith, Donald Spence, Ernesto Spinelli, Sandra Strine, Ercy Soar, Karl Tomm, Angelica Tratter, Ulrike Willutzki, Stan Witkin, and Paul Wholford.

Yet, there are five individuals to whom I owe a special debt of gratitude. Earlier in my career, by invitation of Claus Bahnson, I served for a number of years on the staff of the Eastern Pennsylvania Psychiatric Institute. Claus was wonderfully helpful in introducing me to research and practice in family therapy. However, it was Harry Goolishian of the Houston-Galveston Institute who invited me to participate most fully in exploring therapy as a process social construction. I gained enormously from this relationship, and his premature death remains a tragedy for me. Most fortunately, however, Harry left to me a rich legacy in the form of his colleague, Harlene Anderson. Harlene has been a catalytic presence in the development of my thinking ever since. Finally, I must single out Mony Elkaim for his enormous contribution to my development. His keen intelligence and warm friendship provided the necessary inspiration to undertake the present work.

At last, I must add my deep gratitude to Mary Gergen, who has been an inspiring interlocutor throughout. Traces of her bright conversation may be found on every page.

Kenneth J. Gergen

Part I

Therapy As Constructive Collaboration

1

Social Construction And Therapeutic Communication

The process of being human is the process of meaning-making.
                                                    Robert Kegan

When attending graduate school I was simultaneously laboring to support a wife and two children. The pressures were considerable and domestic relations were deteriorating. The time seemed ripe for a good therapist. It was to him that I began to pour out my thoughts and feelings about the various pressures, complexities, strivings, fears, and passions pulsing through my life. However, not many weeks passed before he seemed to tire of hearing about such matters. Rather, he began directing all his questions to family relations during the early years of my life—to my father's authority, sandbox squabbles with my brother, the shock of seeing my mother naked. After several more weeks it was I who began to tire. Why were we spending countless hours in a distant past when the complexities of the present were so anguishing? Why was his view of what is important in my life more knowledgeable than mine, especially given the relatively short period of acquaintance? Why should he rely on the doctrines of a 19th century Austrian in wrestling with the issues confronting me in the 20th century? Indeed, why should we be focusing on "my problems," dynamics locked within my brain as opposed to byproducts of stressful conditions? Was my therapist not presuming that I was psychologically impaired in some way? Why was I "impaired," rather than "valiant" or "resourceful?"

These early doubts set in motion career-spanning concerns with the theory and practice of psychotherapy and its attendant conceptions of mental illness. My academic work as a social psychologist nicely lent itself to this continuing interest. Early in my career Claus Bahnson invited me to affiliate as a Research Scientist with the Eastern Pennsylvania Psychiatric Institute. Years later I was invited by the ground-breaking therapists, Harry Goolishian and Harlene Anderson, into an especially productive dialogue on issues of discourse and psychotherapy. These inquiries were later enriched many-fold by relations with the many therapist/scholars to whom appreciation was extended in the Preface. My work was also enriched by extended encounters in various institutes and organizations—especially the Houston-Galveston Institute, the Kensington Consultation Centre, DISPUK, The East Side Institute, Fundacion Interfas, and the Family Institute of Geneva.

Yet, in looking back on my early misgivings about the therapeutic process, I have also come to realize that I was scarcely alone. In fact, I have come to see that my early questioning was part of a major sea-change taking place within the scholarly and therapeutic community, one in which honorable traditions were everywhere being thrown into question. In an important sense, the present volume springs from the ashes of the growing doubt in universalized conceptions of truth, objectivity, rationality, progress, and moral principle. All too often such concepts have functioned to impede the generative flow of human relationship. Too often they have been used to constrain the nature of our expressions, and to separate those allowed to participate in determining our collective future from those who are silenced. And too, such conceptions have now contributed to the establishment of a range of self-rationalizing hierarchies of privilege. This is so in the world of psychotherapy no less than other walks of life.

It is from these ashes of doubt that new dialogues have emerged, new voices of hope and promise for human existence. These conversations now move across continents and cultures, and are accompanied by a profusion of professional practices—in therapy, education, social work, counseling, organizational development, conflict resolution, community development and more. There are many names for this revolution in thought and practice. Terms such as postmodernism, post-foundationalism, post-empiricism, post-structuralism, and post-Enlightenment and are often among them. Some speak in terms of a "linguistic turn," and others of a "cultural turn" in our understanding of knowledge and the self. Yet, many of the central ideas move about an orbit usefully characterized as *social constructionist*. In this sense, social constructionism is not a singular and unified theory. Rather, it is better seen as an unfolding dialogue among participants who vary considerably in their logics, values, and visions. While there is substantial sharing, there is no single slate of assumptions to which all would adhere. Indeed, to establish a final truth, a foundational logic, a code of values, or a slate of practices would be antithetical to the very unfolding of meaning championed by the movement.

Many therapists are quite familiar with the landscape of social constructionist thought. Indeed, many have contributed significantly to its development. However, for those presently joining these explorations, some preliminary words may be helpful. Specifically, my attempt in this initial chapter is first to sketch out a series of assumptions shared by many engaged in constructionist explorations. More detailed accounts can be found elsewhere.[1] After describing some of these central ideas, I will take up the challenge of therapeutic communication. Here I will move beyond existing accounts to demonstrate what might be called the *radical relationalism* that constructionism invites. In this context, I shall offer an initial glimpse into the practical implications of social constructionism for therapeutic practice.

The Social Construction of the Real and the Good

There are many ways to tell the story of social constructionism. Some would trace its history back in time to the works of Nietzsche, Goethe, or Vico. Others would focus on more recent developments in the sociology of knowledge or the history of science. In my book, The Saturated Self, I described a growing consciousness of construction emerging from the multiple realities and moralities made evident to us through modern technology. Each of these accounts would, indeed, construct constructionism in a different way, each useful in a different context. In what follows I will move in none of these directions. Rather, I shall briefly describe a number of the most widely shared arguments and proposals circulating today. I have selected four particular themes because they are simultaneously among the most unsettling and profoundly liberating. As the volume proceeds, we shall explore the implications and manifestations of these ideas in therapeutic practice.

The Social Origins of Knowledge

Perhaps the most generative idea emerging from the constructionist dialogues is that what we take to be knowledge of the world and self finds its origins in human relationships. What we take to be true as opposed to false, objective as opposed to subjective, scientific as opposed to mythological, rational as opposed to irrational, moral as opposed to immoral is brought into being by historically and culturally situated groups of people. This view stands in dramatic contrast to two of the most important intellectual and cultural traditions of the West. On the one hand is the tradition of the individual knower, the rational, self-directing, morally centered and knowledgeable agent of action. I shall say more about this concept of self as the volume unfolds, but for now it is important to recognize that the constructionist dialogues challenge the individualist tradition, and invite an appreciation of relationship as central to human well-being. It is not the individual mind in which knowledge, reason, emotion and morality reside, but in relationships.

The communal view of knowledge also represents a major challenge to the view of Truth, or the possibility that the accounts of scientists, or any other group, reveal or approach the objective truth about what is the case. In effect, propose the constructionists, no one arrangement of words is necessarily more objective or accurate in its depiction of reality than any other. To be sure, accuracy may be achieved within a given community or tradition—according to its rules and practices. Physics and chemistry generate useful truths from within their communal traditions, just as psychologists, sociologists, novelists, and priests do from within theirs. But from these often competing traditions we cannot locate a transcendent truth, a "truly true." Any attempt to determine the superior account would itself be the outcome of a given community of agreement.

As you can imagine, these arguments have provoked strong and sometimes angry reactions among scientific communities in particular. Let's say you have devoted a lifetime to pursuing what you believe to be objective knowledge, and you despair of the unverifiable myths, credos, and folk beliefs by which common people lead their lives. Under these conditions it is difficult to be told that science is itself a social construction, and not intrinsically superior to other traditions. Yet, it is my view that such anguish is based on a misreading of the constructionist message. Western medical science, for example, does indeed offer useful truths; most of us would scarcely wish to abandon them. However, these truths are based on an enormous array of culturally and historically specific constructions, for example, about what constitutes an impairment, health and illness, life and death, the boundaries of the body, the nature of pain, and so on. When these assumptions are treated as universal—true for all cultures and times—alternative conceptions are undermined and destroyed. To understand death, for example, as merely the termination of biological functioning would be an enormous impoverishment of human existence. The point is not to abandon medical science, but to understand it as a cultural tradition—one among many.

Thus, social constructionism first serves an enormous liberating function. It removes the rhetorical power of anyone or any group claiming truth, wisdom, or ethics of universal scope—necessary for all. In contrast, for most constructionists, all voices may justifiably contribute to the dialogues on which our futures depend. At the same time, to understand all knowledge claims as socially constructed is not to render them false or insignificant. Again, it is to recognize that each tradition, while limited, may offer us options for living together. In this way constructionism invites a posture of infinite curiosity, where every tradition may offer us riches and new amalgams that stand ever open to development. When we recognize that the realities of today depend on the agreements of today, enormous possibilities are opened. We are not destined to repeat the past; with collaborative innovation new futures are born.

The Centrality of Language

Many scholars believe that Ludwig Wittgenstein was the most significant philosopher of the 20th century. After reading his later work, most especially the Philosophical Investigations, one can never see the aim of philosophy in the same way again. Why? In large measure because Wittgenstein's work challenged the capacity of philosophy to yield true understanding of knowledge, rationality, ethics, the self, and all the other subjects of longstanding concern. As Wittgenstein proposed, our descriptions and explanations of the world are formed within language, or what he calls "language games." Games of language are essentially conducted in a rule-like fashion; to make sense at all requires that one play by the rules. The rules of grammar present the most obvious case; but there are also myriad rules of content. For example, it is not acceptable for me to say that "my love is oblong." The utterance is grammatically correct, and there is no way it can be falsified by empirical data. Rather, our ways of talking about love in the 21st century do not happen to include the adjective, "oblong." Expanding on this point, we can see the major questions asked by philosophers as language games. For example, the longstanding question of whether the mind truly has access to the external world—the "problem of epistemology" as it is called—is a problem only within a given game of language. To play the game we must agree that there is a "mental world" on the one hand and a "material world" on the other (an "in here" and "out there"), and that the former may possibly reflect the latter. If you do not agree to play by these rules, there is no "problem of individual knowledge."

Yet, to view language as simply a game within itself is limited. As Wittgenstein proposed, language use is lodged within broader "forms of life," as he called them. Consider the form of life we call a "soccer match." To be sure, there are traditional ways of talking about soccer—about teams, scores, penalty kicks and so on. But these forms of talk are embedded within forms of action and a material surrounds. One cannot simply yell out, "Score!" on a busy street corner, without rousing suspicion. There are only specific conditions in which such a cry makes sense, and this depends on a specific array of objects (such as the playing field and the ball) and people (such as the players and referees).

Such ideas are highly congenial with the view of knowledge as social in origin. As people coordinate their actions a major outcome is often a system of signals or words. The words often serve to name the world for the participants. This is "a goal," you have a "depression," that is "a mammal," and so on. Yet, as readily appreciated, these words are enormously important to sustaining these relationships. Not only do they represent the agreements regarding what exists for the participants, but they essentially constitute the glue by which their very forms of life—or traditions—

are held together. What sense is there in a jury trial without a language of guilt and innocence; what would the profession of psychology be without a language of the mind; and what would become of religion if we abandoned the language of the spirit?

In this context we realize the enormous power that inheres in transforming language use. When we can alter the ways in which language is used, develop new forms of talking, or shift the context of usage, we sew the seeds of human change. At the same time, we can appreciate deep-seated grounds of resistance.

The Politics of Knowledge

Social constructionism shares much with a pragmatic view of knowledge claims. That is, traditional issues of truth and objectivity are replaced with concerns with practical outcomes. It is not whether an account is true from a god's eye view that matters; rather we ask about the results for our lives that follow from taking any truth claim seriously. There can be many truths, depending on community tradition, but as the constructionist asks, what happens to us—for good or ill—as we honor one as opposed to another account? There are no meaningful words without consequence. In this sense, the increased awareness of the communal construction of the real and the good does far more than unsettle our traditional beliefs in truth, objectivity and knowledge—beyond history and culture. Thrown into question is also the right of any particular group—scientific or otherwise—to claim ultimate authority of knowledge.

Such a conclusion has had enormous repercussions in the academic community and beyond. This is so especially for scholars and practitioners concerned with social injustice, oppression, and the marginalization of minority groups in society. If communities create realities (facts and good reasons) congenial to their own traditions, and these realities are established as true and good for all, then alternative traditions may be obliterated. Regardless of whether we are speaking of scientific fact, canons of logic, foundations of law, or spiritual truths, as we formulate the world we implicitly favor certain ways of life over others. Thus, for example, the scientist may use the most rigorous methods of testing intelligence, and amass tomes of data that indicate racial differences in intelligence. However, to presume that there is something called "human intelligence," that people differ in their possession of this capacity, and that a series of question and answer games reveal this capacity, is all specific to a given tradition or paradigm. Such concepts and measures are not required by "the way the world is." Most importantly, merely entering the paradigm and moving within the tradition is deeply injurious to those people classified as inferior by its standards. Or to put it another way, the longstanding distinction between *facts* and *values*—objective reflections of the world, and subjective desires or feelings of "ought"—cannot be sustained.

As we see, sensitivity to the politics of the real and the good invites a broad critical posture. We may ask of all claims to knowledge, wisdom, insight, and the like, "what follows," "who benefits," and "who is silenced?" Unfortunately, however, many of those drawn into a critical posture simply remain there. The gadfly never becomes a butterfly. To understand the politics of knowledge also opens the door to appreciation. It is not simply "what we lose" within any tradition of knowledge that is important, but what we gain as well. All constructions will place limits upon our lives; but without construction there is nothing worthy of any pursuit. In my view, constructionism invites us all into a dialogue concerning the openings and closings which we inherit from the past. Moreover, to underscore an earlier theme, it is through such dialogues that we are invited to create new orders of intelligibility. From these new amalgams we may move toward richer and more inclusive forms of life.

From Self to Relationship

As earlier discussed, the constructionist dialogues shift our attention from the individual actor to coordinated relationships. The drama here is substantial. Consider: If you were asked to describe your family, chances are you would begin to talk about the various family members. You might describe the differing personalities of a father or mother, perhaps a brother or sister. You might also describe your feelings about each of them, and the impact they have on your life. This common way of describing one's family is revealing: how quickly and unproblematically we assume that the group is made up of independent beings, each with particular characteristics, private feelings, and perceptions of each other. Much the same kind of account would be given of a classroom, a community, or life in an organization. The unspoken and unexamined assumption is that individual actors form the basic atoms of social life. Each of us acts according to internal dictates—of cognition, emotion, motivation, and so on. Each of us is responsible for his or her own actions.

Yet, as the constructionist proposes, all that we take to be real, true, good, valuable and desirable emerge from a process of coordination. The same may be said about our distinction between "me" and "you." The vocabulary of individual minds is not required by "the way things are," nor is the belief in fundamental independence. The conception of human beings may vary dramatically across both culture and history, and even in Western culture the preeminent status of the individual self is of recent historical vintage. Prior to the 16th century, the common individual was typically identified in terms of the group to which he or she belonged— the family, clan, or profession. That the conception of individual selves is constructed is not in itself a criticism. In fact, many of our most precious traditions—democracy, public education, protection under the law—draw their rationale from the individualist tradition. However, to recognize the historical and cultural contingency of individualist beliefs does open the door to reflection. Should we settle for the status quo?

As many argue, there is substantial dark side to constructing a world of individual agents. When we make a fundamental distinction between self and other, we create a world of distances: me here and you there. We come to understand ourselves as basically alone and alienated. We come to prize autonomy—becoming a "self made man," who "does it my way." To be dependent is a sign of weakness and incapacity. To understand the world as constituted by separate individuals is also to court distrust; after all, one never has access to the private thoughts of others. And if alienated and distrustful, what is more appropriate than "taking care of number one?" Self gain becomes an unmitigated virtue—indeed for the economist, an unavoidable rational calculus—until the ethicist comes along and pleads that we "love the other as the self." Loyalty, commitment, and community are all thrown into question, as all may potentially interfere with "self-realization." Such are the views that now circulate widely though the culture.[2] We may not wish to abandon tradition of individual selves, but constructionism invites us to explore and create alternatives.

Movement toward a relational understanding of human action is now gaining momentum, and new practices are emerging in many quarters. On the conceptual level, theorists from many different perspectives are attempting to articulate a vision of a *relational self*. For example, as psychoanalytic theory has shifted toward "object relations," therapists have become increasingly concerned with the complex relations between transference and counter-transference. No longer is it possible to view the therapist as providing "evenly hovering attention," for the therapist's psychological functioning cannot be extricated from that of the client.[3] Family therapists have begun to appreciate the power of shifting from individual narratives to narratives of relationship.[4] From a separate quarter, many developmental theorists and educators are elaborating on the implications of Vygotsky's early view that everything within the mind is a reflection of the surrounding social sphere.[5] From this perspective there are no strictly independent thought processes, as all such processes are fashioned within particular cultural settings. Stimulated by these developments, cultural psychologists now explore forms of thought and emotion indigenous to particular peoples.[6] Discursively oriented psychologists add further dimension to relational theory by relocating so-called "mental phenomena" within patterns of discursive exchange. For example, rather than viewing memory, attitudes, or repression as processes "in the head" of the single individual, they are reconceptualized as relational phenomenon. We come to speak, then, of "communal memory," attitudes as positions within an argument, and repression as an outcome of circumscribed conversation.[7] My own orientation to therapeutic communication, to be treated shortly, is closely allied with such work.

Coupled with these developments in theory are myriad experiments in relational practice. Indeed, many of these experiments are the result of innovations within the therapeutic profession. We shall explore these more fully as the volume unfolds. However, the enrichment of practices in the therapeutic domain runs parallel with developments in numerous other professions. To touch on but a few, research methods in the social sciences are undergoing a profound change, as scholars increasingly seek ways of bringing those who are traditionally the "objects of study" into productive dialogue with the researcher. Participatory action research represents a full flourishing of such attempts, as the researcher works with various individuals or groups to effect needed change.[8] In the educational sphere, we find a growing investment in collaboratively oriented classrooms, relational bonds between teacher and student, collective performance, and dialogic forms of pedagogy.[9] Organizational development specialists now search for means of reducing the gap between "leader" and "follower," and conceptualizing leadership as a particular configuration of relationships.[10] Practices of top-down organizational change are replaced with group deliberation and collaborative meaning making.[11] Additional practices centering on relational process may be found in the spheres of community development, social work, and conflict reduction.[12]

It is important to realize that this explosion of relational theory and practice does not simultaneously cast out what has preceded. Unlike traditional orientations to knowledge, constructionism does not attempt to eliminate previously existing ideas and practices. There is no reason to silence any tradition. Rather, the invitation is to expand on what is available to humankind. Thus, traditional experimental research and statistical analysis is not abandoned, nor old fashioned lecturing, or charismatic leadership. Rather, constructionism invites us to see the limits of these traditions, and to expand our dialogue and enrich our practices in ways that are congenial with a relational perspective.

These four themes—centering on the social construction of the real and the good, the pivotal function of language in creating intelligible worlds, the political and pragmatic nature of discourse, and the significance of relational process as opposed to individual minds—have rippled across the academic disciplines and throughout many domains of human practice. As you can appreciate, all such developments are controversial. The interested reader may wish to explore the various critiques and their rejoinders.[13] However, such ideas also possess enormous potential. They have the capacity to reduce orders of oppression, broaden the dialogues of human interchange, sharpen sensitivity to the limits of our traditions and to their potential offerings, and to incite the collaborative creation of more viable futures. Such is the case in therapy as it is in the global context.

The therapeutic community has long participated in the constructionist dialogues. As early as 1993, Sheila McNamee and I edited a volume, Therapy as Social Construction, a volume that went on to be translated into several languages and to enjoy a happy life within enclaves of family therapy in particular. This volume brought into common dialogue the voices of systemic, narrative, constructivist, and brief therapists— among others—and suggested a broad sea-change in thought and practice. I will have much to say about this transformation in subsequent chapters. However, to set the stage for these explorations it will be very helpful to explore a single issue in more detail. Specifically I would like to focus on the process of therapeutic communication. The process is of singular significance, not only to the outcomes of therapy but to the very idea of a constructed world. This discussion will also help to clarify differences between constructionism and contrasting traditions, and to appreciate its profoundly relational character. After treating some of the rudiments of the communication process we can turn to specific applications to therapeutic practice.

Therapeutic Communication Reconsidered

Effective therapy often seems magical. A life shattering problem is described in the quiet recesses of a chamber far removed from the site of turmoil. Questions and answers, stories good and bad, emotional outbursts, a little silence and perhaps some tears—all may ensue. And then, almost by miraculous intervention, there is change. The problem is transformed, seems less severe, or is possibly dissolved. Yet, we ponder, how was the result achieved? What is it about this particular configuration of events that brought about change? At least one central candidate for answering this particular form of "miracle question" is therapeutic communication. There is something about the nature of communicative interchange that engenders change. Yet, to answer in this way is scarcely sufficient. How are we to understand the process of communication? What precisely is it about communication that brings about transformation? What forms of communication are invited; how might we be more effective?

These issues are scarcely new. They have been focal from the time Freud laid out the logic of interpreting the unconscious, to the groundbreaking work of Watzlawick, Beavin and Jackson (1967). Nor is the challenge posed by these questions simply one of theoretical nicety—an

academic exercise of little consequence. Rather, conceptions of therapeutic communication lie somewhere toward the center of practice.
Whether rudimentary or conceptually rich, our assumptions about communication inform and insinuate themselves into all therapeutic practices.
Consider the client who complains of his lack of sexual desire. If you are
a marital counselor, you are likely to treat these words as an accurate
representation of reality, and set out to offer a program of support. In
contrast, if you are a psychoanalyst you are likely to disregard the client's
account of his life, and to use his words as messages from a world off-
stage, namely the domain of the unconscious. For the constructivist therapist, however, the same words are neither descriptions of the real world
nor manifestations of repressed desires, but indicators of the world from
the client's perspective. The therapist might thus launch inquiry into the
logic of this perspective, its possible distortions, and the like. And, for the
structuralist family therapist, the client's words may be understood in
none of these ways, but as indications of the configuration of family relations. In this case the therapist might address the ways this expressed lack
of desire is related to the actions of other family members. Each presumption about the nature of language and the process of communication
yields a different therapeutic posture.

In what follows I wish first to consider several major assumptions
that underlie most therapeutic practices developed to date. Although there
is much to be said on behalf of these assumptions, in each case I wish to
single out major shortcomings. While our conceptual heritage is rich, our
traditional assumptions about therapeutic communication occlude our
vision and erect barriers beyond which our practices cannot proceed. I
shall begin to lay out the rudiments of a constructionist theory of communication. In this account we find a dramatic disjunction with the past, a
shift to a radical relationalism. I want finally to consider some specific
implications for therapeutic practice. As we explore a new view of the
communication process, so do we generate new sensitivities and open
new options.

Traditions in Trouble

The therapeutic community inherits an estimable tradition of thought regarding the nature of communication. At the same time, this tradition now comes under increasing criticism—both by therapists attempting to place it in action and scholars exploring its conceptual structure. Let us briefly consider several traditional assumptions and the critical problems they create:

The Realist Assumption. One of the most broadly shared views of language is based on the assumption that words are (or can be) reflectors of the real. That is, language can (and should) function so as to provide accurate accounts of what is the case. This is the view inherited by most of the sciences, as they set out to replace misleading, fallacious or superstitious beliefs with true and accurate accounts of the world. For many therapists it is also essential to distinguish between client accounts that are accurate, realistic and truthful, vs. those which are distorted, fanciful, or duplicitous. The realist assumption is also central to those attempting to develop diagnostic categories and measures of pathology. In daily life it is a view that lends support to the distinction between objective facts and subjective opinions, and moral weight to demands that people "tell the truth."

There is much to be said about the importance of this tradition both to scientific and cultural life. However, as the preceding discussion makes clear, the realist assumption is deeply flawed. There is no privileged relationship between a given language and the state of things; there is no particular arrangement of words and phrases that is uniquely tailored to the "world as it is." Rather, as we have seen, declarations of the real and the true are always located within relationships—friendships, families, communities, traditions. Within these relationships there can be undisputed realities—"myocardial infarction" in medicine, a "three point shot" in basketball, and so on. In this sense, to tell a lie is not to misrepresent the world, but to violate a communal tradition.

The Subjectivist Assumption. Often coupled with the realist assumption is a second view of longstanding. As it is typically said, we each exist in our own private worlds of experience, a mind set apart from, and reflecting upon nature—a state of subjectivity that variously reflects conditions of the objective world. On this account, the words we speak are held to be outer expressions of the inner world, the subjective mind made manifest. This view has played a major role in science, as we count the scientist's words to reflect his or her experience of the world, and demand that observations be shared to insure agreement among subjectivities ("objectivity" as shared "subjectivity"). The assumption is critical to most all therapy of the past century, save perhaps to the radical behaviorist methods of the 1950-60s. In almost all cases we listen to a client's language as an outer expression of private experience (or, as in the Freudian case, that which lies beneath conscious experience to give it shape). And, the assumption is a common feature in daily relations, as we speak of the difficulties in knowing what others mean by their words, or how they "really feel." Intimacy, we believe, is a reflection of the closeness of two otherwise independent subjectivities.

Here I shall only touch briefly on the problems of subjectivity. Two such problems are focal, the first conceptual and the second ideological. On the conceptual level, it is important to realize that no one has yet been able to give a defensible account of how a person's words give us access to his or her inner world. Given another's utterances, we have no way of knowing what they say about the speaker's subjective state. Hermeneutic theorists, concerned with how it is we can accurately understand the intentions behind the words of the Bible or holy writs , have worried about the problem of "inner access" for over three centuries now. A satisfactory answer to this question has never been forthcoming. In Hans Georg

Gadamer's (1975) pivotal work, the major emphasis shifts to the "horizon of understanding" which the reader inevitably brings to the text. As Gadamer reasoned, all readings must necessarily draw from this forestructure of understanding—what it is the reader presumes about the world, the writing, the author, and so on. And reading must inevitably take place from this horizon. Much the same conclusion is reached by a host of "reader response" theorists in literary studies. As Stanley Fish (1980) has put the case, every reader is a member of some interpretive community, a network of people who understand the world in certain ways. And whatever interpretation of the text is made, will inevitably rely on these understandings. In effect, the reader never makes authentic connection with the subjectivity of the writer; there is no escape from the standpoint one brings to the interpretation.

The dismal conclusion of this line of criticism is that we never gain access to the other's subjectivity; we never understand each other! We shall revisit this problem shortly. However, there is a second line of attack on the subjectivity assumption, one that resonates with our earlier discussion of the politics of knowledge. Here it is variously proposed that by placing such importance on individual subjectivity we give further support to an individualist ideology, an ideology detrimental to our cultural future. To reiterate some of the earlier critiques, when we hold individual subjectivity as the essential ingredient of humanity, we simultaneously construct a world of fundamentally isolated individuals, each locked within their own private world. All we have to count on, ultimately, is ourselves. Others are by nature alien, and because self-seeking is the obvious choice under such conditions, others may indeed be seen as potential enemies. When the quality of individual subjectivity is paramount, all forms of relationship—marriage, friendship, family, community—are necessarily artificial and secondary. If this form of ideology retains its pervasive grip on cultural life, the future seems grim. In effect, the subjectivist assumption is socially corrosive.

The Strategic Assumption. There is a third problematic assumption regarding communication, one often made by therapists in particular. It is frequently held that communication operates as the major means by which individuals influence each other's actions. More specifically, it is reasoned, each of us uses language to achieve our goals, satisfy our desires, etc. Because of the complexities of daily life, we must rationally consider what we can say, when, where and to whom. Language typically functions, then, as a strategic implement through which we achieve their goals. It is in this sense, as well, that the therapist may select his/her words carefully, insert them into the conversation at the proper juncture in order to change to client or the pattern of family relations.

In light of the preceding discussion, the problems of the strategic assumption require but brief attention. For one, the position borrows heavily from the subjectivist tradition—"I desire and plan, and therefore I speak." In this sense, the strategic assumption suffers from the same conceptual enigmas and the ideological shortcomings just discussed. Private goals are preeminent; others become secondary, mere utilities in the service of self. When we play out the implications of the strategic assumption the critique is intensified. When we understand communication as primarily serving private ends, human relations become a sea of manipulation. When we view communication in this way, acts of trust seem naive, commitment a sign of weakness, and the pursuit of human rights little more than a political ploy. Even the therapist undermines his/her credibility, as the motive behind his or her communication to the client becomes suspect The therapist may be viewed as a master manipulator and clients may come to see themselves as mere pawns. A strategic orientation can be fractionating.

Communication as Coordinated Action

In my view, there is a significant transformation taking place in many sectors of the therapeutic community. There is broad discontent with traditions that presume the existence of an unconscious, of mental illness, of specifically individual problems, and the assumption of value neutral knowledge. Many therapists are dismayed by the standardization therapeutic techniques, diagnostic manuals, and mechanistic models of individual or family functioning. Many therapists are also quite willing to abandon the realist and the strategic orientations toward communication, and entertain doubts in the mind as the source of human action. There is an increasing concern with the significance of communal meaning making, the constructed nature of reality, co-constructive processes in therapy, and the cultural and political character of therapeutic practice. Issues of narrative, metaphor, problem definition and dissolution, and multiple realities are topics of lively discussion. In effect, a constructionist sensibility is already pervasive in many therapeutic quarters.

The question that must now be asked is whether an alternative conception of human communication can be hammered out, one that is at once more catalytic and congenial with such movement. Can such a conception avoid repeating the problems inherent in the earlier traditions? My belief is that a new view of human communication can indeed be drawn from the constructionist dialogues, not only as they are taking place within therapeutic circles but as they have developed in the neighboring domains of ethnomethodology, the history of science, the sociology of knowledge discursive psychology, literary theory and communication theory.[14] In each of these cases there is a strong tendency to place the locus of meaning within the process of interaction itself. That is, the individual agent is de-emphasized as the source of meaning; attention moves from the *within* to the *between*.

Although recognition of the jointly constructed character of meaning has become increasingly widespread, there is as yet no comprehensive account of how such a process occurs. If we accept such an orientation, what are the action implications; what new conceptual resources can be mobilized, what new questions are raised? For purposes of furthering the dialogue, in what follows I shall make a preliminary incursion into these domains. I offer here a series of rudimentary propositions that place meaning squarely within the relational matrix:

An individual's utterances in themselves possess no meaning.

We pass each other on the street. I smile and say, "Hello Anna." You walk past without hearing. Under such conditions, what have I said? To be sure, I have uttered two words. However for all the difference it makes I might have chosen two nonsense syllables. You pass and I say "Umlot nigen..." You hear nothing. When you fail to acknowledge me in any way, all words become equivalent. In an important sense, nothing has been said at all. I cannot possess meaning alone.[15]

The potential for meaning is realized through supplementary action.

Lone utterances begin to acquire meaning when another (or others) coordinates themselves to the utterance, that is, when they add some form of supplementary action (whether linguistic or otherwise). Effectively, I have greeted Anna only by virtue of her response. "Oh, hi, good morning..." brings me to life as one who has greeted. Supplements may be very simple, as simple as a nod of affirmation that indeed you have said something meaningful. It may take the form of an action, e.g. shifting the line of gaze upon hearing the word, "look!" Or it may extend the utterance in some way, as in "Yes, but I also think that...." We thus find that to communicate at all is to be granted by others a privilege of meaning. If others do not treat one's utterances as communication, if they fail to coordinate themselves around the offering, one is reduced to nonsense.

To combine these first two proposals, we see that meaning resides within neither individual, but only in relationship. Both act and supplement must be coordinated in order for meaning to occur. Like a handshake, a kiss, or a tango, the individual's actions alone are empty. Communication is inherently collaborative.

In this way we see that none of the words that comprise our vocabulary have meaning in themselves. They are granted the capacity to mean by virtue of the way they are coordinated with other words and actions. Indeed, our entire vocabulary of the individual—who thinks, feels, wants, hopes, and so on—is granted meaning only by virtue of coordinated activities among people. Their birth of "myself" lies within relationship.

Supplementary action is itself a candidate for meaning.

Any supplement functions twice, first in granting significance to what has preceded, and second as an action that also requires supplementation. In effect, the meaning it grants remains suspended until it too is supplemented. Consider a client who speaks of her deep depression; she finds herself unable to cope with an aggressive husband and an intolerable job situation. The therapist can grant this report meaning as an expression of depression, by responding, "Yes, I can see why you might feel this way; tell me a little more about your relationship with your husband." However, this supplement too stands idle of meaning until the client provides the supplement. If the client ignored the statement, for example going on to talk about her success as a mother, the therapist's words would be denied significance. More broadly, we may say that in daily life there are no *acts in themselves*, that is, actions that are not simultaneously supplements to what has preceded. Whatever we do or say takes place within a temporal context that gives meaning to what has preceded, while simultaneously forming an invitation to further supplementation.

Acts create the possibility for meaning but simultaneously constrain its potential.

If I give a lecture on psychoanalytic theory, this lecture is meaning-less without an audience that listens, deliberates, affirms, or questions what I have said. In this sense, every speaker owes to his or her audience a debt of gratitude; without their engagement the speaker ceases to exist. At the same time, my lecture creates the very possibility for the audience to grant meaning. While the audience creates me as a meaningful agent, I simultaneously grant to them the capacity to create. They are without existence until there is an action that invites them into being.

Yet, it is also important to realize that in practice, actions also set constraints upon supplementation. If I speak on Freud, as an audience member you are not able to supplement in any way you wish. You may ask me a question about object relations theory, but not astrophysics; comment on the concept of repression but not on taste of radishes. Such constraints exist because my lecture is already embedded within a *tradition of act and supplement*. It has been granted meaning as a "lecture on Freud," by virtue of previous generations of meaning givers. In this sense, actions embedded within relationships have *prefigurative* potential. The history of usage enables them to invite or suggest certain supplements as opposed to others—because only these supplements are considered sensible or meaningful within a tradition. Thus, as we speak with each other, we also begin to set limits on each other's being; to remain in the conversation is not only to respect a tradition, but to accede to being one kind of person as opposed to another. If you tell me that I have not been a good friend, I will scarcely be recognizable unless I ask you to tell me why you feel this way, and what have I done. Your very comment constrains my potentials.

Supplements function both to create and constrain meaning.

As we have seen, supplements "act backward" in a way that creates meaning of what has preceded. In this sense, the speaker's meaning—his or her identity, character, intention, and the like—are not free to "be what they are," but constrained by the act of supplementation. Supplementation thus operates *postfiguratively* , to create the speaker as meaning this as opposed to that. From the enormous array of possibilities, the supplement gives direction and temporarily narrows the possibilities of being. Thus, for example, for a therapist, to inquire into a client's depression is to establish a form of constraint. If the client is to remain sensible, he or she may readily accede to being depressed. A therapeutic question can harbor implications for an entire life trajectory.

While act/supplements are constraining, they do not determine.

As proposed, our words and actions function so as to constrain the words and actions of others, and vice versa. If we are to remain intelligible within our culture, we must necessarily act within these constraints. Such constraints have their origins in a history of preceding coordinations. As people coordinate actions and supplements, and come to rely on them in everyday life, they are essentially generating a way of life. If enough people join in these coordinated activities over a long period, we may speak of a cultural tradition. Yet, it is important to underscore that our words and actions function only as *constraints*, and *not as determinants*. This is so for two important reasons: First, the conditions under which we attempt to coordinate our actions are seldom constant. We are constantly faced with the challenge of importing old words and actions into new situations. As we do so, such words and actions acquire new possibilities for meaning. For example, you are visiting a farm and you point out to your child, "look...that is a chicken." The word "chicken" thus gains its meaning from the way it is embedded in this configuration of events. Later that day, the farmer's wife comes to the dinner table bearing a large platter, and announces, "We are having chicken for dinner tonight." Now the word used in referring to the live and clucking animal refers to the individual pieces of cooked meat. As new situations develop, so will the same word acquire other potentials for meaning. More formally, we say that all words are *polysemic*;" they may be used in many different ways.

A second important reason for our relative freedom of action lies in the fact that meaning making is always local. That is, coordination is always located in the here and now, in momentary and fleeting conditions—in the kitchen, the boardroom, the mine, the prison, and so on. These local efforts to coordinate give rise to local patterns of speaking and action—street slang, academic jargon, baby talk, jive talk, signing, and so on. And, because those who enter into such coordinations may issue from different cultural traditions—new combinations are always under production. In effect, we inherit an enormous potpourri of potentially intelligible actions—each arising from a different form of life—and the repository is under continuous motion. Our actions may be invited by history, but they are not required. In this sense, we can indeed "step over our shadows," and in order to function adequately in continuously changing circumstances, creative combinations will always be necessary. As we speak together now we have the capacity to create new futures.

Traditions of coordination furnish the major potentials for meaning, but do not circumscribe.

To amplify a preceding line of reasoning, it is important to recognize that the words and actions upon which we rely to generate meaning together are largely byproducts of the past. If I approached you and began to utter a string of vowels, "ahhh, ehhhh, ooooo, uuuu...," you would surely be puzzled; perhaps you would make for an exit, as I might well be dangerous. This is so because this utterance is nonsense, or to put it another way, not recognizable as a candidate for meaning within Western traditions of coordination. Similarly, if we began to dance and you suddenly crouched and gazed at the floor, I would scarcely continue dancing. Your actions are not part of any coordinated sequences with which I am familiar. Our capacity to make meaning together today thus relies on a history, often a history of century's duration. We owe to traditions of coordination our capacities for being in love, demonstrating for a just cause, or taking pleasure in our children's development.

This is not to say that there is no room for novel words and actions. Indeed, in the past century we have witnessed an explosion in new vocabulary terms, sporting activities, dance steps, and so on. Because we are not determined by the past, we are free to play, to violate expectations, to explore the outrageous. And, when we confront the novel word or act, we can with effort bring it into meaning. To return to our dance, I might well stop dancing when you crouched on the floor. However, if I understood you to be playing, inviting, challenging, I would do my best to find a means of coordinating with you. Perhaps I would also crouch, and begin to sway forward in your direction...Thus, an adolescent who wears something "weird" to school may give rise to a fad. And therapists who believe the Schizophrenic's "word salad' is meaningful will find ways to render such utterances meaningful.

Thought and feeling consist of public meaning making conducted privately.

As offered earlier, we do seem to experience what might be call "private meaning." If an intimate friend expresses anger toward us, we may lapse into silence, unable to respond. However, this does not mean that the word has no meaning to us. A dozen replies may buzz through our head; we ride an emotional roller-coaster. Let us not deny the significance of such an event. However, the existence of unspoken replies does not simultaneously mean a reinstatement of the subjectivity assumption, the view that meaning originates in private minds and is expressed outwardly in words. We must avoid the problems inherent in the view that there is an internal agent inside who can rise above cultural meaning, who possesses the capacity to generate meaning prior to any immersion in a relational world. Let us, rather, reconstruct the meaning of subjectivity—the "inner world." Consider: you have agreed to take part in a play, and you must master your lines before tonight's rehearsal. With the script before you, you speak the lines; when they are familiar you put the book down and perform them more fully...perhaps with a laugh or a shout. You decide to take a shower, and while you are showering you try to recall the lines silently. During the silent rehearsal you move through a clever line and a smile crosses your face. You "feel" the mirth. Here we see that the distinction between the internal and external world breaks down. What takes place internally is essentially an action in the public world, only conducted without full expression. The internal activity is effectively a reduced form of making sense in our common relationships. As some scholars put it, thought is a form of internal speech—a public act simply carried out in private.

In much the same way, we may usefully reconfigure the concept of intention. We commonly speak about our intentions as causing our actions. For example, we say to ourselves, "I must apologize," and then we proceed to do so. To be sure, the apology may not be defined that way by others; in this sense I need them to make it an apology. However, I did know what I was doing at the time, from my perspective, and this knowing *preceded* the supplementation. Such common events are often used to support the assumption of conscious agency: I chose my actions, I intend certain meanings and not others. This concept of a free, internal agent that directs the traffic of one's words and deeds has a long tradition, and much contemporary support from humanistic scholars. Yet, in spite of its attraction ("I am the god of my action..."), the concept has faired poorly both philosophically and ideologically. The notorious problem of free will on the one hand, and the politics of narcissism on the other, are only two of the knotty issues. How can we sustain the conception of conscious intention without falling into these traditional traps?

We find a promising answer by extending the view of thought and feeling as the private recirculation of public life. If I am an actor who does what we call, "playing the part of Hamlet," I can readily tell someone that, "I am playing Hamlet tonight." Public life provides me then with a pattern of action and an acceptable construction of that action. It allows me to tell others that "this is what I will do." Of course, I may silently say this to myself as well, as in: "Hmmm...I really shouldn't take this drink...I will be playing Hamlet tonight." These private constructions— resulting from my participation in public life—are what we may call intentions. They do not direct the action so much as comment upon its occurrence. In this way I can say, "I intended that remark as an apology..." I can say this with full assurance, because my immersion in public life gives me grounds for knowing that the words I have uttered are commonly defined as an apology. By the same token, we can say, "he intended to commit the murder," not because we have insight into his conscious state, but because his experience in cultural life furnished him with just this construction of the act in question.

Meanings are subject to continuous reconstitution via the expanding sea of supplementation.

In light of the above, we find that what an utterance means is inherently undecidable. No amount of discussion, discourse analysis, conversation analysis, or other attempt to determine what has been said, can be determinative. The meaning of any utterance is a temporary achievement, born of the collaborative moment. Further, as relations continue over time, what is meant stands subject to continuous alteration through an expanding arena of action/supplements. Sarah and Robert may find themselves frequently laughing together—affirming each other as humorous persons—until Robert announces that Sarah's laughter is "unnatural and forced," just her attempt to present herself as an "easy going person" (in which case the definition of the previous actions would be altered). Or Sarah could announce, "this is all very pleasant, Robert, but really you are a superficial guy; we really don't communicate at all." (Thus reducing Robert's humor to banality). At the same time, these latter moves within the ongoing sequence are subject to further reconstitution (In reply to Robert's accusation of being unnatural, Sarah replies, "Robert, are you worried about your job again? What's bothering you?" Or, Robert replies to Sarah's ascription superficiality with, "Now I see...You are only saying that, Sarah, because you find Bill so attractive.") Such instances of alteration may also be far removed from the interchange itself (e.g. consider a divorcing pair who retrospectively redefine their entire marital trajectory), and are subject to continuous change through interaction with and among others (e.g. friends, relatives, therapists, the media etc.).

In summary, we find the exclusive focus on the face-to-face relationship is far too narrow. For whether "I make sense" is not under my control; nor is it determined by you, or the dyadic process in which meaning struggles toward realization. At the outset, we largely derive our potential for coordination from our previous immersion in a range of other relationships. We arrive in the relationship as extensions of the past. And, as the current relationship unfolds, it serves to reform the meaning of the past. These interchanges may be supplemented and transformed by still others in the future. In effect, meaningful communication in any given relationship ultimately depends on an extended array of relationships, not only "right here, right now," but how it is that you and I are related to a variety of other persons, and they to still others—and ultimately, one may say, to the relational conditions of society as a whole. We are all in

this way interdependently interlinked—without the capacity to mean anything, to possess an "I"—except for the existence of an extended world of
relationship.

Therapy as Collaborative Action

Developed here is a particular way of understanding the process of communication from which meaning emerges, is sustained and transformed.
This account avoids certain pitfalls of most traditional accounts, and simultaneously realizes some of the potentials of constructionist reasoning. It is important to point out that I am not saying that, "now we know
the true nature of communication." Rather, this view is offered in the
spirit of constructionism itself: it is simply an alternative way of making
communication intelligible. The question is not whether it reveals the
"reality of communication," but what follows from such an exposition?
In what way would such an understanding alter any of our practices, and
would such alterations be useful for the therapeutic venture? To be sure,
such questions cannot be answered all at once. There are many implications, both great and small, and further dialogue is needed to glimpse the
potentials and problems. Some of the implications of this collaborative
account are already well integrated into practice; other implications will
prove too radical for contemporary application. However, to open discussion on therapeutic communication as collaborative action, I offer the
following nine points:

1. There is no mental anguish or illness in itself.
    Because no human expression comes into meaning save through oth-
ers' supplements, there is no suffering and no mental illness prior to collaboration. To be sure, I may "feel depressed," or encounter an "obvious
schizophrenic." But the fact that I feel depressed is already prepared by a
previous immersion in a culture of circulating meaning. (Prior to the 20th

century I could not "feel depressed," because the very intelligibility of depression only emerged within this century.) In the same way we "see schizophrenics," because are already participants in a culture that collaborates to create the meaning of "mental disease." I will go into some of the socio-political implications of this view in Chapter 4. However, for now it is important to lay stress on the responsibilities of the therapist in creating and/or sustaining the life of anguish and illness within the therapeutic relationship. The therapist functions as a major collaborator in the generation of meaning; whether the client is anguished or ill, resourceful or resilient, is importantly dependent on the continuing collaborative process.

2. There is no therapeutic treatment in itself.

If the therapist bears some responsibility for how clients come to understand themselves, their feelings, their relationships and so on, this is not to say they are omnipotent in their effects. For their supplements are also actions in themselves, and in this sense, do not acquire meaning until supplemented by the client. To put it more broadly, there is no "therapeutic treatment" in itself; the actions that we might normally describe as "therapeutic treatment" do not become so until clients are willing to collaborate with this view. Custodians in mental hospitals know this very well. Often their honest attempts to help patients yield anger and resentment. Good treatment from the custodian's perspective is manipulation and control from the patient's. We must ask, then, whether we should reconsider what we as professionals call "good treatment." If the concept of "good treatment" is not collaboratively generated, then positive outcomes are unlikely.

3. Therapeutic understanding is a form of collaborative action.

We inherit a psychological view of interpersonal understanding. As we say, understanding occurs when subjectivities are linked or reflect each other accurately. Earlier we located important flaws in this view. As argued, if understanding were a matter of inter-subjective synchrony, we would never understand each other. Yet, we do believe that understanding occurs, and we are certain when another misunderstands us. How can we account for understanding from the collaborative view?

Here it is useful to view understanding not as a mental activity, but as a particular form of supplementation. To be "understanding" is to coordinate one's actions to those of another; it is to be a certain kind of person in relation to the other. It is a coordination of words, gaze, posture and so on with the other's actions. Perhaps the major form of action is captured by the term, metonymy. Formally, *metonymy* is a term from semiotics, referring to the use of a single word or phrase to stand for the whole. For example, the flag of France is sometimes used to stand for the nation as a whole, or a crown is displayed as the symbol of the queen of England. In an important sense, our actions may also carry metonymical reflections of each other. If you speak to me with humor about an incident, and I respond with a broad smile, I am now carrying a part of you. My smile is a small symbol of you, now expressed by me. If another speaks of their anguish, a listener "understands" when part of this anguish is then carried in his or her reply. If the listener simply gazed out the window during the tale of sadness, the speaker might justifiably say, "You just don't understand, do you?" There is no peering into the mind of the other here; there is only coordinated action.

4. Therapeutic change derives from collaborative action.

What is actually changed through therapy? Consistent with its individualist base, this question is typically answered in terms of the individual psyche. It is through the removal or repression, a process of catharsis, a gain in insight, the enhancement of self-esteem, or the alteration in cognitive schemas, as it is variously reasoned, that long term change is effected. From the present perspective the landscape is dramatically altered. The psychological condition is not the center of concern but relational existence. The individual arrives in therapy as a participant in a relational network, a network that extends outward from intimates to culture at large, and backward in time to preexisting relationships and traditions. It is this matrix of relationship out of which "the problem" is created and designated as a problem. The therapeutic relationship represents the establishment of a new coordination, a coordination that will develop from the resources that both the therapist and client bring to the relationship. The major challenge confronting the therapeutic relationship is whether the collaborative trajectory of client/therapist can unsettle or transform the generative matrix in such a way that the problem is resolved, dissolved, or reconstructed.

In this sense we see that the therapist's most valuable resources are conversational actions. In the same way that skilled basketball players possess a rich vocabulary of actions enabling them to score, so are skilled therapists those who are able to coordinate effectively with the client in such a way that agreeable outcomes may be achieved within the extended matrix. It is not the storehouse of facts, concepts, distinctions and so on that the therapist has at his or her disposal that counts, but the capacity for flexibility in relationship. "Knowing how" as opposed to "knowing that." This relational capacity will surely be verbal. Required are capacities to move in narrative, metaphor, exploration, irony, humor, pathos, curiosity, imagination and much more. Yet, it is not simply the language content that is important. Posture, gaze, tone of voice, facial expression, gait, and so on all contribute to the form and ramifications of relationship. All may be used to unsettle or transform the matrix. All may provide the client with models for action outside the therapeutic relationship.

Because therapy is inherently a coordination, and no two clients will enter from the same relational matrix, there can be no hard and fast rules for the therapeutic encounter. Specific techniques or canons of therapeutic practice will only narrow the capacities for coordination. If the client recognizes the therapist's utterances as "technique," they may indeed be disregarded or resented. Thus, there is no unequivocal answer to the question of "how should I proceed?" The same words and phrases useful in one context may be crippling in another. Again the basketball analogy is useful: with experience the skilled player develops a repertoire of usable actions. There are no rules for which action is most effective; the conditions of play are complex and rapidly changing. The skilled player is one who can rapidly draw from the repertoire as the "conversation of the court" unfolds. A skilled player can "unsettle" the opponent's "traditions of action." At the same time the opponents will also model these skills and become more proficient. The patterns of play continue to unfold. In the case of therapy, there are no opponents; there is only the collective construction of well-being at stake.

5. The major resistance to therapeutic change may not be present.

When working with a concept of meaning as relational coordination there is a strong tendency to stress the here and now—"us talking together at this moment." It is in the present moment that meaning is under construction, and thus the future in the balance. Yet, this focus often obscures the ways in which the resources imported into the therapeutic session are anchored in relational history. This history can stand as a major impediment to change. On the simplest level, people develop modes of talking and acting that are comfortable and reliable. In an important sense, they are skilled in these forms of action. Thus, depressive, angry or self-critical styles of being may seem dysfunctional from the therapist's standpoint. However just such modes of action may serve as reliable, "natural," and finely honed skills for the client. "I know so well how to attack others for their shortcomings," a client may say. "Even if others avoid me for this reason, this is what I know how to do." Without new skills or performance capacities in hand, a client may scarcely relinquish the old.

On a more subtle level, all of us carry with us residues of past relational patterns. As proposed earlier, it is the private recirculation of these residues that we speak of as "thought" or "emotion." Such forms of recirculation may establish themselves as recurring scenarios. There is the voice, for example, that says, "You are no good," and a following one that gives you a lift, "Yes you are, you are great!" You perform with the latter voice at hand and things go well. The cycle repeats, and you develop what might be called a private "coping scenario." Such privately recirculated scenarios may not always be so functional, as in "You are no good...I will hurt you for saying that...but everybody agrees that you're no good...I will fight them all..." Performances predicated on such a scenario may be suspicious and hostile. These privately recirculated and well-worn scenarios may be the most difficult to interrupt. Anyone who has worked with what we commonly label as "eating disorders" has encountered the strangulating grip of the private conversation. In my view one of the most challenging problems confronting contemporary therapy is that of linking the face-to-face conversation with the client to the off-stage scenarios.

6. Therapeutic revelation is not movement in vertical but in horizontal space.

Often therapy is viewed as a revelatory process, one in which the therapist's probing questions lead to the revelation of that which is otherwise concealed. "Ahaa...now we know what is truly troubling you..." In effect, we find much therapy based on a view of surface vs. depth—that which is up front and conscious, vs. that which lies hidden beneath. Although psychoanalytic therapy is the most obvious case in point, such a view is widely shared within the culture at large. We readily speak, for example, of people who are "shallow," of expressing "true feelings," and of "the real reason he wants this..." However, from the present perspective we find that the very idea of "surface" vs. "depth," is a collaborative achievement. That is, we have together created this particular view of persons. It is essentially optional.

This is to say that there is no principled reason for "probing the depths" of a client's desires, memories, or motives. The therapist in such instances is inviting the client into a relationship in which "depth" will be created as a conversational object. Such "depth discourse," is not more profound in implication than "surface discourse;" it is simply creates a different reality within the therapeutic setting. I am scarcely proposing that we should thus abandon the discourse of depth. Rather, it is to raise the question of its efficacy within any given case. What does the creation of a "reality behind the reality" accomplish within the client's existing patterns of understanding? Are the client's existing ways of talking discredited; are new avenues opened by this kind of talk; what are the possible consequences? The recent crises in therapeutic authority resulting from the wave of "child abuse memories" produced in the therapeutic hour adds dimension to such questions. The important question is not whether therapeutic collaboration "hits the nail on the head," with respect to the client's problems or past, but whether the nail may subsequently injure someone's head.

7. Every statement about meaning is a transformation in meaning.

From the collaborative perspective, each move within a conversation grants meaning to what has preceded. The meaning of all our words and actions is importantly dependent on those who respond to them. And their responses are denied significance until they too are supplemented. In effect, meaning is always in process, never complete, forever open to the next move in the conversation. This is to say that any attempt to specify the meaning of a past action—"what I intended..." "what I was trying to say..." "what you did to me..." "what this meant to me..."—

is itself a supplement that transforms the past. Such attempts give the past shape and consequence that could not be acquired save through the attempt itself. And these attempts as well stand mute until supplemented. There is no final moment of illumination, a moment at which meaning becomes indelible and undeniable.

The therapeutic implications of this reasoning are many. First, and to underscore an earlier argument, any therapeutic interpretation of a client's words or actions create the meaning of those words and actions. Any attempts by the therapist to point out continuities or discontinuities within the client's life, are themselves creations of continuity and discontinuity. Further, any attempt by the client to speak about the past, to reveal its secrets, to render it meaningful is itself a transformation of the past. Amplifying Donald Spence's (1982) arguments, this is to make prominent the significance of narrative as opposed to historical truth. Accounts of the past are created within the conversational space of the present.

It also follows that all attempts at psychodiagnostic testing and therapeutic outcome assessment, are essentially transformations of meaning. In both cases, whatever has occurred, whatever has been said or done, is granted a certain meaning that it did not itself possess. There is no pathology until the testing instrument has transformed the individual's words and actions into pathology. There is no positive or negative outcome of therapy until the assessment device renders certain patterns meaningful as outcomes. Important questions must thus be addressed: for whom is this pathology, what makes this diagnostic category more useful than another; are illness categories useful for clients; who is deciding on what constitutes a "good outcome," what clients and therapists are benefited (or marginalized) by a given conception of outcome; whose voices are allowed into the conversation; and when does the conversation terminate? In effect, from the view of communication as coordination, the practices of diagnosis and outcome assessment should be opened to full reexamination.

8. Therapy may be a wonderland; the important question is actionability.

If we follow the collaborative logic, therapy represents a conversation in which participants borrow heavily from their relations outside, but in which they simultaneously create the grounds for a new and unique reality (discourse patterns shared by them alone.) Under these conditions it might be possible for therapist and client to locate a wonderfully agreeable mode of relating—a shared sense of harmony and fulfillment within the encounter. However, this same reality may also be wholly contained within the relationship. That is, it may have little or no "street value," little transportability into other relations. Given the collaborative view, the major question is whether the conversational resources generated within the therapeutic relationship are actionable outside this context. Can the metaphors, narratives, deconstructions, reframings, multiple selves, expressive skills and so on developed within the therapeutic encounter be carried into other relations in such a way that these relations are usefully transformed?

At one level, I have little doubt that such reverberations do occur. However, more effective demonstrations of the ways in which the therapeutic conversations or discourses actually insinuate themselves into the life worlds of clients would be very useful. Further, more concerted attention is needed to how the two contexts—therapy and life world—can be made to converge. The most obvious means, and one very congenial to the family therapy movement, is to work with relationships rather than single individuals. In this way new discursive forms and practices are set directly in motion. However, this does not fully solve the problem, as the group reality of the therapeutic hour may not be transportable; family members are also embedded in multiple relationships outside the family circle. The family in the therapy room is not the same family at the dinner table.

9. Therapeutic practices must be continuously transformed.

For over a century now, therapists have searched for "the cure" to the problems confronted by their clients. It is thus that we have witnessed a parade of therapeutic schools, each eager to champion their particular form of treatment, and typically dismissing the remaining field of contenders. In the U.S. there are longstanding attempts to assess the comparative efficacy of various practices, thus to winnow out the "mere pretenders." In other nations the laws only recognize a narrow range of schools as worthy of health insurance coverage; the remaining are left to perish.

When we understand meaning as collaboration, we open a new chapter in this discussion. Every therapeutic school contributes to the discursive resources of the culture. Their distinct moves in the collaborative process of meaning making offer possible departures from convention. In this sense, the plethora of therapeutic schools is not an embarrassment—somehow an indication of the pre-scientific status of the field. With the immense variations in cultural history from which clients emerge, we must cease to think in terms of a "master conversation," useful to all. Rather, we have here a case in which multiple realities are to be valued.

To extend the argument, we must also recognize that therapeutic schools are themselves self-sustaining traditions. Typically they tend to reaffirm a particular vocabulary and honor certain moves in conversation over others. In this sense schools of therapy become culture-conserving. Yet, while the internal discourses of a school remain stable, the meaning making process within the culture continues to spin on. New forms of coordination (and dis-coordination) are everywhere in motion. Today's profundity becomes tomorrow's platitude. Passions are cooled and values forgotten in the continuously unfolding illuminations generated by active and creative dialogue. In this way we see that we can never settle for the existing family of therapeutic schools. All are endangered by irrelevancy. Rather, we must support the continuous evolution of therapeutic language and practice. It is when therapeutic conversations are continuous with those of the culture that they will most effectively "make sense." It is when the client can coordinate the discourse of therapy with his or her life outside that therapy is most likely to succeed. New schools of therapy should not only be anticipated, but welcomed.

Let us bring the discussion to a temporary end. In the preceding pages I have sketched the contours of what many see as major transformations in our understanding of truth, objectivity, rationality, morality, and progress. As traditional assumptions are challenged, we leave the moorings of the "individual self" and give ourselves over to the continuous flow of relational being. Here we found that all communication depends on relational coordination, and that individual sense-making represents but an extension of the coordination process. In this light, the questions we ask of therapy take on a special hue. Many traditional issues slip from sight, their relevance now impugned. New issues emerge, new challenges, and new possibilities. We are prepared, then, for the more detailed excursions of the following chapters.

2

Therapeutic Practice
As Social Construction

*If I were to wish for anything, I should not wish for wealth and power,
but for the passionate sense of the potential...what wine is so spar-
kling, so fragrant, so intoxicating, as possibility!*

Soren Kierkegaard

As we pass into a new century we are witnessing a gradual but ever inten-
sifying convergence in conceptions of the therapeutic process. At the heart
of this convergence lies the human activity of generating meaning. First
and foremost we find the therapeutic relationship one in which human
meaning is not only focal, but pivotal to the process of therapeutic change.
Significant preparation for the contemporary movement has come from
many sources, including humanistic/phenomenological/hermeneutic psychologists have long argued for the centrality of individual meaning to
the therapeutic process; the pioneering work of George Kelly (1955) and
the ensuing dialogues on constructivism (cf. Neimeyer and Mahoney,
1995) have also placed individual construal at the center of the therapeutic relationship. The emergence of object relations theory in psychoanalytic circles further stressed the interdependence of meanings within family
relations and between the therapist and client (Asbach and Schermer, 1987;
Mitchell, 1995); the work of the Palo Alto group—eventuating in
Watzlawick, Jackson and Beavin's classic, <u>Pragmatics of Human Com-
munication</u>—extended this emphasis on interdependent meanings within
families; Milan systemic therapists carried this orientation forward into a
range of new and challenging practices.

As these early dialogues on meaning have unfolded and interacted the therapeutic community has become increasingly open to the vortex of critical and constructionist interchange within the broader intellectual community. The result has been a persistent though uneven shift toward a common conception of meaning—away from its traditional locus within individual minds to its creation within relationships—from mental to social construction.[16] For some the shift is subtle and adjustments are minor; however, in its more radical form this transformation does nothing less than subvert all existing foundations of therapeutic thought and practice. To be sure, this movement has provoked a substantial degree of antagonism (cf. Held, 1996; Sass, 1992; Mancuso, 1996; Lannamann, 1998). More productively, however, a range of significant questions has emerged: what, if any, are the significant threads uniting these diverse movements; are there important differences; in what important ways does a constructionist shift disrupt existing therapeutic traditions; should we anticipate or hope for singular mode of treatment; how are these orientations to be reconciled with traditional investments in diagnosis and mental health policies; what is being lost in this transformation and what is gained?

It is from this context of ferment and self-reflection that I shall first attempt to extricate a number of pivotal assumptions playing through the emerging dialogues on construction, to sharpen them through comparison with existing traditions, and to treat some of the central problems which they raise. This will be to illuminate and clarify a family of interlocking assumptions to which many therapists now subscribe in varying degrees. The attempt is not to generate a new foundation for therapy, nor a canonical formulation of "postmodern therapy;" both these goals would be antithetical to social constructionist dialogues. Rather, the hope is that the present discussion can contribute to generative conversation, a maturing of sensibilities, and the emergence of new practices. This latter aim will become particularly focal in the last section of this chapter. Here I will outline a heuristic means for enriching therapeutic practice.

Social Construction and Therapist Orientation

I wish first to focus on four transitions in understanding that follow from a conception of therapy as the relational construction of meaning. While these transitions have a variety of practical implications, my focus here is not centered so much on specific techniques as the kind of therapist sensitivities that are invited. What do these shifts in assumption invite in terms of our thinking about therapeutic options? Consider the following:

From Foundations to Flexibility

Traditional orientations toward therapy are derived from what are commonly viewed as rational foundations of knowledge. These foundations are typically lodged within what is narrowly defined as an empiricist conception of knowledge. As this tradition has played out in the social sciences, most professionals have come to hold that theories of human behavior should be grounded in observation. With continued and rigorous observation we should approach a true and objective understanding of both normal and abnormal behavior. Further, from this standpoint, continued research should reveal which of a variety of therapeutic practices is most effective for treating various forms of abnormality. There may be many candidates for truth about persons, dysfunctions, and cure, but empirical research should, on the traditional account, ultimately enable us to winnow the many to a few—and ultimately to perhaps one.

For the social constructionist theories of human action are not built up or derived from observation, but rather grow from our collective attempts to interpret the world. In this sense, it is the conventions of intelligibility shared within one's professional enclave that will determine how we interpret the observational world. Thus, a psychodynamic therapist will find evidence for repressed desires, while a cognitive therapist will locate problems in the individual's mode of information processing, and a family systems therapist will be drawn to the realities of family communication patterns. Because theories serve to construct the world in their terms, there is no means of empirically testing between them. Each "test" would inevitably construct the field of relevant facts in its terms and thus serve to privilege some theoretical standpoint as opposed to another. Outcome research is subject to the same problem; a positive outcome from one therapeutic standpoint (e.g. symptom reduction, expressed feelings of well-being) may signify a regression or problem exacerbation for others. From certain standpoints even suicide may be counted as a positive outcome.

Based on this line of reasoning constructionism invites an abandonment of the search for foundations—a single view of knowledge or human functioning that prevails over all others. The constructionist dialogues encourage us to relinquish the longstanding competition among schools of therapy, along with the related conceptions of fixed diagnostics, "best practices" of therapy, and outcome comparison. Rather, if we view the various therapeutic schools as communities of meaning, then each school possesses transformational potential. Each offers an opening to a form of life. Lynn Hoffman (1985) captures much the same idea in her view of theories in family therapy. For her, theories, "represent sets of lenses that enforce an awareness that what you thought looked one way, immutably and forever, can be seen in another way. You don't realize that a 'fact' is merely an 'opinion' until you are shocked by the discovery of another 'fact' equally persuasive and exactly contradictory to the first one. The pair of facts then presents you with a larger frame that allows you to alternate or choose. At the cost of giving up moral and scientific absolutes, your social constructionist gets an enlarged sense of choice." (p. 4)[17] Similarly, Cecchin, Lane and Ray (1992) write, "Having too much faith in any position, any story, we run the risk of creating an inflexible, impoverished therapeutic reality, (which is why) we pose the question, how can we train ourselves to be disloyal to any story when or if it becomes no longer useful." (p. 14)

The major implication of this line of reasoning for therapeutic practice is clear: the therapist is invited to move across the domain of therapeutic intelligibilities and practices and to employ whatever may be serviceable in the immediate therapeutic context. In this sense, there is no "social constructionist method" of therapy. To formalize any method—to canonize its principles—is to freeze cultural meaning. It is to presume that effective processes of forging meaning in the present will remain so across time, circumstance, and context of interpretation. This is also to say that the common critique of the therapeutic community—that the multiple and ever shifting field of theory and practice reveals a state of confusion and a lack of real knowledge—is ill founded. This very richness of intelligibility and the capacity of the therapeutic community continuously to refashion understanding represent perhaps its most significant strength.

Yet, the implications of this position are more radical than that of favoring of theoretical and practical eclecticism. Within the empiricist tradition the professional account of the person and the therapeutic process was privileged over that of the common culture. Whereas the quotidian understandings of the culture were said to be fraught with bias, misunderstanding, and superstition, the discourse of the profession furnished more comprehensive and accurate understanding. For the constructionist the criterion of "more accurate or objective understanding" is removed; all forms of understanding are culturally embedded constructions. Effective therapy may—and typically will—require the use of many speech genres, including those of the culture at large. This is to say that for purposes of therapeutic practice, the door is opened to the full range of cultural meanings. To be sure, this may include all existing forms of therapy—from psychoanalytic, behavior modification, cognitive, Rogerian, and more.

At the same time, we must be prepared to radically expand the arena of usable meanings. For example, there is strong support here for those wishing to include spiritual discourse within the therapeutic process (see for example, Griffith and Griffith, 1992; Richards and Bergin, 1997; Butler, Gardner and Bird, 1998). For much of the population such discourse speaks in a powerful way; to neglect its significance is therapeutically myopic. However, the complete therapist should not shun the discourses of romance, New Age, Marxism, Zen Buddhism, and more. The skilled therapist in a constructionist mode might be as much at home speaking the language of the street, the locker room, or the night club as mastering the nuances of Lacanian analytics. Each new intelligibility enriches the range and flexibility of the relational moment.

We should not conclude from this analysis, however, that professional theories are without special merit. Professionally developed theories are especially significant in their capacity to offer alternatives not easily located within the common culture. Therapeutic theories represent enormously important innovations in making human action intelligible. In this sense the culturally deviant theory of the professional may possess unique generative power. In deviating from common sense it may significantly challenge the status quo, shake the cage doors of conventionality, and offer genuinely new directions of inquiry. Further, professional languages enable therapists to engage in communal deliberations—to speak meaningfully with each other and thus to coordinate their efforts more effectively. Such discourse further enables the therapeutic community to reflect critically on the common intelligibilities of the culture—which reflection cannot be done from within these intelligibilities themselves. The culture critiques of Erich Fromm, Karen Horney, and Herbert Marcuse are illustrative.

Similarly, the abandonment of foundations does not mean the end of inquiry into therapeutic outcomes. Every outcome—from reducing alcohol consumption, domestic violence, or depression to that of creating a sense of personal growth or consciousness of archetypes—reflects a tradition, a way of life, or a tradition of value. The point, then, is not to abandon traditional modes of valuing. Rather the more profitable path is to 1) expand on the range of value considerations taken into account in any outcome (e.g. broaden consideration on what may count as a positive or negative outcome), and 2) set in motion dialogues in which competing and conflicting values or outcomes may be discussed. By taking into account multiple criteria of "wellness" we not only expand the domain of what it means to be fully functioning, but generate a more differentiating and reflective picture of what counts as "the healthy person," when, and for whom.

From Essentialism to Consciousness of Construction

As suggested the modernist therapeutic tradition is invested in truth. Thus, therapy is typically oriented toward locating "the real problem," the "causes of the difficulty," "the forces at work," "the determining structures," and the like, and assessing the effects of contrasting therapeutic practices on outcomes. For the constructionist there are no problems, causes, forces, structures and so on that do not derive their status as such from communally based interpretations. This is not to propose that "nothing exists," or that "we can never know reality,"—common misunderstandings of constructionism—but rather that when we attempt to articulate what exists, to place it into language, we enter the world of socially generated meanings. It may be more helpful, then, to say that constructionism operates against the tendency to essentialize the language, that is, to treat the words as if they were pictures, maps or replicas of essences that exist independent of we who interpret our existence in this way. In effect, constructionism serves as a continuous reminder of Gregory Bateson's dictum, "the map is not the territory."

Of course, the proclivity of therapists to point out ways in which clients' accounts of self and world fail to match the territory has been a professional mainstay since Freud's pioneering work on repression. Ever since, therapists have been alerted to the client's possible failure to properly appraise "the real world." However, until recently most schools of therapy have presumed both the existence of the territory of "the real," and the function of words as mapping agents. It is only under these assumptions that such terms as "delusion," "distortion," "misperception," and "misattribution," are intelligible. Constructionism, in contrast, invites us to see such terms in a horizontal rather than a vertical plane, that is, as indicators of an alternative way of constructing the world (one among many) as opposed to the necessary or superior way. To accuse a person of being deluded is primarily to say that he or she does not share your interpretive conventions. Early movement toward the horizontal plane can be found in the work of the Milan school, and particularly the practice of circular questioning. The importance of circular questions in this context is that it does not represent an exploration of "what is the case" in the family, but rather attempts to generate information that can make a difference in the shared understanding of family members (Selvini-Palazzoli, et al, 1980). A circular question such as "Father, which of your two children do you think your wife is closest to, Vicki or Joe?" does not function to illuminate the truth about family structure, but rather to bring forth possible ideas that might challenge the problematic logic shared by the family. A similar attempt to replace essentialism with a consciousness of construction is evident in brief therapy, and particularly the work of de Shazer (1993, 1994). As Berg and de Shazer (1993) propose, "Meanings arrived at in a therapeutic conversation are developed through a process more like negotiation than the development of understanding or an uncovering of what is 'really' going on." (p. 7)

This emphasis on constructed realities must be accompanied by an important caveat. Constructionism does recognize the significance of truth in context. Within any community there will be tendencies toward essentializing the commonly shared modes of discourse—treating the language as a "map of the real"—and this essentialization is of inestimable importance in sustaining the community's traditions. We may name this infant Diana and that one David, and while the names are arbitrary the essentializing moves (e.g. It is true that, "Diana is my daughter" and "David is at school.") are necessary to maintain the local orders of family, school, friendship, and so on. Similarly, while the language of biology is not required by "what exists," agreement on the way in which the language of genes and chromosomes is used within the profession is essential for what we call "in vitro fertilization" and "DNA testing."

This is also to say that consciousness of construction does not necessarily invite therapists into a posture of deconstructing client realities. Effective therapy does not require ontological crisis, and indeed, is more often likely to leave most of the client's understandings intact. As Harlene Anderson (1997) puts it, "My role as a therapist is to participate with a client in a first-person linguistic account of his or her relevant life events and experiences." (p. 114); similarly, Tom Andersen (1991) writes, "If people are exposed to the usual they tend to stay the same. If they meet something un-usual, this un-usual might induce a change. If the new they meet is very (too) unusual, they close up." (p. 19) Consciousness of construction is most valuable as an orientation that invites the suspension of reality during those times in which the taken-for-granted or essentialized reality proves painful or problematic. If a client's "problem" seems intractable then the deconstruction of existing narratives or accounts of the real may be an essential precursor to reconstruction.

From Expertise to Collaboration

As proposed, there is no singular set of practices that follow or can be derived from a constructionist view. For example, there is nothing about constructionism that would necessarily be against the therapist's "taking an authoritative stand" in a therapeutic relationship; strong and directive opinions may sometimes be useful. However, if we play out the implications of constructionism as a theory of human action, new doors are opened to practice. In particular, constructionist theory invites the therapist to consider alternatives to the traditional position of authority, and particularly to explore a collaborative orientation to the client. The shift in style is no small undertaking. As Hoffman (1993) writes, "the change from a hierarchical to a collaborative style...is a radical step. It calls into question the top-down structuring of this quasi-medical field called mental health and flies in the face of centuries of traditional western practice...To challenge these elements is to challenge the whole citadel." (p. 4) As Tom Andersen (1995) describes his therapeutic work, it has moved toward "heterarchy." "Hierarchy governs from the top and down, and heterarchy governs through the other...More common words for a heterarchical relationship might be 'democratic relationship,' an 'even relationship,' or a relationship with equally important contributors." (p. 18)

More controversially, in their "collaborative language systems" approach, Anderson and Goolishian (1992; Goolishian, 1992; Goolishian and Anderson, 1997) proposed a collaborative partnership with the client in which the therapist enters with a stance of "not knowing. "Not-knowing refers to "an attitude and belief that a therapist does not have access to privileged information, can never fully understand another person, always needs to be in a state of being informed by the other, and always needs to learn more about what has been said or may not have been said...Interpretation is always a dialogue between therapist and client and not the result of predetermined theoretical narratives essential to a therapist's meaning, expertise, experience or therapy model." (Anderson, 1997, p. 134) This is not to say that the therapist does not bring uniquely valuable skills to the relationship. It is to say, however, that such skills are not derived from a mastery of descriptive and explanatory accounts of therapy. They are primarily skills in knowing how as opposed to knowing that—of moving fluidly in relationship, of collaborating in the mutual generation of new futures.

Many therapists moved by this vision look with disfavor toward traditional, strategic options. More generally, strategic interventions are seen to be monologic (as opposed to dialogic), dictated by the therapist's private standpoint—developed either in advance of or silently during the therapeutic session. For the collaborative specialist, such strategic action is not only manipulative, but generates a sense of inauthentic participation in the therapeutic relationship (e.g. the therapist's reality is off-stage). In our view, these reactions are not entirely warranted. Again, nothing is necessarily ruled out by constructionism, and surely no one would wish to abandon deliberation on what courses of action are best. Thus, rather than abandoning the strategic orientation, we might opt for dialogues of difference, that is, discussions of how and why strategic intervention can be advantageous and under what conditions it is problematic. Consider, for example, amalgamated orientation that may be termed *situated strategy*. Here the therapist may bring to the relationship multiple logics of action, no one of which is decided in advance. However, as the therapeutic relationship unfolds, various logics might be placed in motion as circumstances invite. Strategic thinking, in this case, is situated—if and when invited by the relationship—and its particular character dictated by the therapeutic relationship itself.

From Value Neutrality to Value Relevance

From the empiricist standpoint therapy is not a forum for political, ideological, or ethical advocacy. The good therapist, like the good medical doctor, should engage in sensitive observation and careful thought, unbiased by his/her particular value biases. Critiques of the assumption of value neutrality have long been extant. The works of Szasz (1970), Laing (1967), and participants in the critical psychiatry movement have made us acutely conscious of the ways in which well intentioned thera-pists can contribute to forces of oppression. Spurred by Foucault's (1979) critique of the "disciplining" effects of therapeutic practices, many recent analysts have focused on ways in which various therapies and diagnostic categories contribute to sexism, racism, heterosexism, individualism, class oppression, and other divisive biases. From a constructionist standpoint even a posture of non-engagement or "neutrality" is viewed as ethical and political in its consequences(Mackinnon & Miller, 1987; Taggart, 1985). Whether mindful or not, whether for good or ill, therapeutic work is necessarily a form of social/political activism. Any action within a so-ciety is simultaneously creating its future.

Many therapists, cognizant of the relationship between therapeutic constructions and societal values, have begun to explore the implications of ethically and politically committed therapy. Rather than avoiding value considerations, socio-political aims become central. We have, then, the development of therapies that are specifically committed, for example, to challenging the dominant order (see for example, White and Epston, 1991) and pursuing feminist, gay, socialist and other political ends. Feminist therapists, for example, frequently focus on female oppression as a fun-damental therapeutic theme, or deconstruct gender categories to provide clients an expanded set of options (Sheinberg, 1992). Social therapy car-ries with it a vision of equalitarian society (Newman, 1991). With the expanding power of identity politics there is every reason to anticipate an expansion in such investments.

Again, while such movements are invited by constructionist dialogues, there is good reason for critical reflection. For we confront here the pos-sibility of an anguished fragmentation—the development of multiple thera-peutic enclaves each claiming a moral high ground, each isolated and righteously attempting to achieve its political aims. Not only would such a condition work against fruitful conversation, but we would approach an antagonistic state in the therapeutic world of all-against-all. In my own view I believe there is inherent in the constructionist dialogues implications for a more positive alternative.

We begin to locate this alternative with the constructionist premise that there are no foundations—no final justifications—for any ethical or political claim. To be sure, to live within any tradition means favoring some values or ways of life over others. In this sense we should scarcely wish to abandon our attempts to create the good society. However, constructionism does remove the ultimate authority of such investments. It removes the foundations for just the kind of commitments that are most frequently used to silence or obliterate those whose voices differ from one's own. And it does invite therapists into mutually transformative dialogue with clients who do not share their views on such matters as abortion, divorce, or physical abuse. In addition, in its emphasis on the ultimate interdependence of all meaning, constructionist arguments suggest a new and different role for therapists. In addition to the options of either avoiding political issues or ardently pursuing social change, therapists are invited to explore the possibilities of bringing disparate groups into coordination, rendering alienated languages more permeable, enabling people to speak in multiple voices, and ultimately reducing the potential for mutual eradication. Value commitment is tempered by practices of co-creation.

Social Construction and Therapeutic Practice

As we have seen, social constructionist dialogues favor four major movements in therapeutic orientation—movements toward flexibility, consciousness of construction, collaboration, and value relevant practice. However, such dialogues also invite a new range of practices. Many of these practices are now well entrenched in certain circles; others are under development. In each case it is important to see their relationship with constructionist thinking. I will focus here on five major shifts in practice:

From Mind to Discourse

Most traditional therapy is focally concerned with individual mental states. From the psychoanalytic emphasis on psychodynamics, Rogerian concerns with self regard, to contemporary cognitive therapy, it is the central task of the therapist to explore, understand, and ultimately bring about transformation in individual minds. Even group psychotherapy has retained a strong investment in psychodynamic principles. As outlined in the preceding chapter, interest in therapeutic communication did begin to occupy increasing attention over the years, and within recent decades converging interests in family systems, communication pragmatics, and second order cybernetics—among the more visible—have brought issues of language into major focus. Yet, as also proposed in the preceding, the constructionist dialogues extend these discussions in significant ways. It is largely through the discursive relationship that realities, rationalities, values and desires come into being, flourish or expire.

This shift to discourse is perhaps the most widely apparent aspect of therapy in a constructionist frame, and has given rise to a broad range of therapeutic innovations. As Sluzki (1992) has put it, therapy may be understood as a process of "discourse transformation." If meaning is generated within linguistic processes, then it is to these processes that attention is drawn (Elkaim, 1997; Kogan and Brown, 1998). The vast share of innovative work has been congenial with the groundswell of social science interest in narrative, or essentially the storied construction of self and world (Bruner,1986; Sarbin, 1988; Polkinghorne, 1984). For many therapists Donald Spence's Narrative Truth and Historical Truth represented a critical turning point. Here was a practicing therapist of long experience who no longer believed that historical truth could be captured in the patient's accounts of his/her early life, and explored the positive uses of the narrative truths developed in therapy.

Yet, perhaps the most prominent expression is found in what McLeod (1997) calls the "postmodern narrative movement." As developed by therapists such as White and Epston (1991) and Hudson and O'Hanlon (1991), and enriched and expanded in numerous ways over the years (Freeman, Epston and Lobovits, 1997; Parry and Doan, 1994; Zimmerman and Dickerson, 1996; Freedman and Combs, 1992; Olver, 1997; McLeod, 1997, 1998; Neimeyer, 1999) the prevailing concern is with the ways in which language constructs self and world, and the implications of these constructions for client well-being. The radical implication of such work is that life events do not determine one's forms of understandings, but rather, the linguistic conventions at our disposal determine what counts as a life event and how it is to be evaluated. It is much the same concern with the force of language in constructing client realities that has sparked the therapeutic use of metaphor (Combs and Freedman, 1990; Schnittman, 1993; Snyder, 1996), and the development of client writing practices as therapeutic tools (Bacigalupe, 1996; Lange, 1996).

Yet, while much has been gained from this watershed, dangers and limitations are also at hand. Four of these deserve particular attention. First, even with an abiding constructionist consciousness, there is a pervasive tendency to objectify discourse, that is to treat meaning as simply "there in nature" as an object of study and transformation. As constructionism warns us, even the concept of discourse is a construction, or in effect, a conversational achievement. It is only when discourse itself (what we take to be a person's narrative or metaphor) can be seen as "one way of putting things" that one gains the freedom to employ alternatives. Practically speaking, there may be instances in which it is more fruitful to treat discourse as, for example, a manifestation of psychodynamic processes or emotional urges. In effect, it is important to sustain the reflexive posture in which even discourse itself may be treated as one reality among many.

Further, there is a continuing tendency to treat discourse as an individual possession, with meaning understood residing in personal consciousness. Indeed, a mainstay of the western tradition is the belief that words are manifestations of meanings that originate within the individual mind. However, this emphasis on personal meaning obscures the constructionist emphasis on language as relational and pragmatic, generated not within but between persons for use in their relationships. Or, for the constructionist, one can never have meaning isolated from relationship. This emphasis on personal meaning is often coupled with a third problem, which is that of treating a change in discourse as equivalent to cure. As often reasoned, if one learns to see life in a different way, to re-narrate the self, or shift from culturally dominant to an individualized conception of self, then improvement has been achieved. Such assumptions not only borrow from the individualist heritage (e.g. "Mental change will produce behavioral change.") but favor as well a view of meaning as a force of its own. In contrast, if narratives and metaphors are forms of discourse, as constructionist writings suggest, then they not so much determine one's actions as they are resources used by people in generating meaning together. If stories are social performances, the we must raise questions concerning the value of a single life-narrative (which diminishes one's capacity for relationship), and the capacity of therapeutically generated narratives to prosper in the social world more generally. We shall return to this issue shortly.

Finally, many of the emerging therapies are limited in their narrow definition of discourse—principally as spoken or written language. Given our traditions this is a comfortable starting point, enriched as well by an expansive literature on semiotics, literary theory, rhetoric, and linguistics. At the same time such a preoccupation is reductionistic. First it reduces discourse to the utterances (or writing) of the single individual. Yet, if meaning is the byproduct of relationship, then such a focus is blind to the relational process from which any particular utterance derives its meaning. In effect, words mean nothing in themselves, and it is only by attending to the flow of interchange that we can appreciate the origins, sustenance and decay of meaning. Further, the emphasis on words strips discourse of all else about the person (and situation) that is essential to generate intelligibility. One speaks not only with words, but with facial expressions, gestures, posture, dress and so on. Ultimately it is important to add bodily and material dimensions to our concern with communication. It is here that constructionism joins hands with many ecologists, sustainability advocates, and wholistic endeavors. With each new addition to our conception of discourse we add to the range of possible practices.

From Self to Relationship

The traditional therapeutic emphasis on mental states is in close harmony with the western belief in the individual actor as the atom of the social world. For at least 300 years we have moved progressively toward what is now simply a taken for granted fact: the individual's public actions are byproducts of internal states of mind (e.g. thoughts, emotions, motives, choice, desire, and memory). Shouldn't therapy, then, be primarily focused on the internal world of the individual? And yet, within recent years we have also become increasingly conscious of the biases built into this view. For example, on the traditional view, relationships are secondary or artificial contrivances, constructed from the raw materials of independent selves. In an attempt to correct for this individualist bias, movements in group and family therapy have offered a range of alternative practices built around such concepts as group dynamics, family structure, and psychological interdependence.

With the constructionist shift from mind to discourse the terrain shifts significantly toward the primacy of relationship. As Wittgenstein (1963) argued, there can be no private language; if you created your own private language you could not communicate. In effect, language is a fundamentally a relational phenomenon—much like a handshake or a tango, it cannot be performed alone. Or in Shotter's (1984) terms, meaning is not created by individuals acting alone, but in joint-action. Or, returning to the thesis developed in Chapter 1, meaning is not located within the mind of individual actors, but is a continuously emerging achievement of relational process. It is in this context that we appreciate more fully the earlier emphasis on co-construction. It is within the relational matrix of therapist-and-client that meaning evolves.

Yet, while many of the practices included in this analysis share this premise, the emphasis on relationship (as opposed to individual mind) expands in many directions. It is useful here to think of concentric circles of relationship, starting first with the therapist-client, and expanding then to the client's relationship with immediate family, intimates, friends and the like. At a first level of expansion, some therapies press backward in time to consider relationships in the distant past. As Mary Gergen (1999) has proposed, we carry with us a cadre of "social ghosts." As one means of tapping into these often significant relationships, Penn and Frankfurt (1994) sometimes ask clients to write letters to a lost loved one. Further expanding the circle, still other therapies take into account the broader community—the workplace, church and the like. In Sweden, Egelund (1997) and his colleagues include in their "town therapy" parents, teachers, social workers, and others whose opinions bear on the putative problem. And finally, other therapies are vitally concerned with the relationship of the individual to the broad social context—to institutions of power, cultural traditions of suppression, and the like. The "social therapy" of Newman and Holzman (1996) , for example, attempts to link individual problems with the broad social conditions of society—race relations, employment opportunities, and community action. In the same vein, Freeman, Epston and Lobovits (1997) write, "Since problem-saturated stories are nested in social, cultural, economic and gender assumptions about roles and behavior, we inquire about these factors and strive to be aware of how they are affecting different family members." (p. 51)

While challenging and innovative, relational practices require continuing attention. There is, for one, the constant danger of reviving metaphors of social determinism, in which the self becomes the byproduct or victim of others—family, occupation, social structure and the like. In effect, the individual must act against others—removing him/herself from their thrall—if success is to be achieved. This tendency toward deterministic conceptions is also invited by the traditional definition of relationship as "an association between or among things." Thus, we tend to consider the individual's relationship with, let's say, his parents or wife, with the individual and the other constituting individual entities. As outlined in Chapter 1, attempts to move beyond this view—placing the relational prior to the individual are extant. However, their flowering is slow. As such views are incorporated into the therapeutic setting, the grip of social determinism may be loosened. Here I like Kathy Weingarten's (1998) view that "I am subject to the same world-making and unmaking processes as everyone else, I can never locate myself as an objective outsider, but must always know myself as a participant." (p. 5)

Finally, it is important here to underscore the anti-totalitarian thrust of constructionism. While the present emphasis is strongly on relational as opposed to intra-individual processes, we should not make the mistake of objectifying the domain of the relational. Relationships should not replace the individual as the "really real." (See also Parre and Sawatzky, 1999) The shift to the relational opens a range of new and practices; however it does not mean abandoning explorations of self—talk about one's emotions, memories, desires and the like. Again, there is nothing about constructionism that argues for the destruction of traditions. Rather, we are invited to see the focus on the self as a cultural tradition, one way of proceeding in therapy and not the only or essential way. Moving outward into the expanding rings of relationship offers additional possibilities.

From Singularity to Polyvocality

Traditional therapies have been enchanted by metaphors of the singular and unified. By this I mean, first of all, that the therapeutic community has gathered round the dream of the single best therapy. We continuously carry out evaluation studies in the hopes of finding which form of therapy is the most effective. Further, we have convinced ourselves that the ideal person is coherent in mind and action. We have not been content with internal tensions, splits, and multiplicities of self. (Consider, for example, the "diseases" of multiple personality disorder and schizophrenia).

With the emergence of constructionist consciousness, the traditional romance with unity is placed in question. The argument for multiple constructions of the real—each legitimate within a particular interpretive community—renders the concept of the "single, coherent truth" both parochial and oppressive. Further, with increasing consciousness of the multiple relationships in which people are embedded—each constructing one's identity in a different way—the ideal of a unified self seems increasingly unappealing. Indeed, in a cultural context of rapidly expanding networks of relationships, the call to singularity also seems counteradaptive (Gergen, 2001). To thrive under these conditions of rapid change may require something akin to a protean personality (Lifton, 1987). It is within this intellectual and cultural context that a new range of therapeutic practices has been nurtured or refashioned.

In this context, many therapists within a constructionist frame press toward multiplicity of client realities. As Weingarten (1998) writes, "a postmodern narrative therapist is generally uninterested in conversation that tries to ferret out the causes of problems. Instead, she is extremely interested in conversations that generate many possible ways to move forward once a problem has arisen." (p. 114) or as Riikonen and Smith (1997) put it, "It would be a mistake to think that inspiring worlds can only be built in one way." (p. 46) It is here that the work of Tom Andersen (1991, 1995) and his colleagues on reflecting process provided an important breakthrough. Using multiple observers of a family, for example, each free to reflect on their interaction in his/her own way, family members are exposed to a range of possible interpretations. Further, as the family is invited to comment on these interpretations, they are set free to consider all options—including those which they develop as alternatives. There is no attempt here to determine the "true nature of the problem," but rather to open multiple paths of interpretation, and thus paths to alternative futures.

In addition to practices of interpretive enrichment, many other therapists have specifically focused on self-multiplicity. Most pointedly, for example, Karl Tomm (1999) has developed a process of "internalized other interviewing," during which his questions draw out the voice of another person within the client. For example, if a client is uncontrollably angry at another person, the client might be asked to imagine him or herself in the other's shoes, and speak from the "position of the other." Can the client find the voice of the other within him or herself; to do so is to bring the anger under control. In a more general frame, Penn and Frankfurt (1994) find that many of their clients enter therapy with "constricting monologues." As therapists, they encourage the development of "narrative multiplicity." They first introduce the possibility of alternative voices—for example positive, optimistic or confident—into the conversations with clients. Then, the client is encouraged to write letters to persons living or dead, dialogues, notes to themselves, journal entries, poetry—in a manner that evokes new voices within themselves. Similarly, Riikonen and Smith (1997) are concerned with the ways in which culturally dominant discourses constrict individual action. Classic are cases of physical or sexual abuse, where victims too quickly embrace conventional views in which they are defined as unworthy or deserving the abuse. In such situations the therapists ask such questions as, "Where do you think these oppressive descriptions come from? Which other types of descriptions/voices in you have been silenced? Have you been able to listen to other ideas? What might it mean if you were able to listen more to those different ideas?" (p. 123) As Hermans and Kempen (1993) further detail, the new voices set in motion internal dialogues that have significant potential for change.

In the Western tradition of singularity in truth and self, this emerging emphasis on multiplicity represents a movement of far reaching consequences. Yet, while enormously rich in implication, we also confront significant questions. In certain respects, to encourage multiple realities is to violate cultural conventions of singular truth, and for many such a move invites a condemnable relativism. If everything is possible, then what has value; what is worth doing? And what of those who long only for "the answer" to their problems; do they now find themselves lost in a vertigo of options? If no option is more reasonable than another, then how is choice possible? It seems clear that like other constructionist practices, pressing toward multiplicity must also be situated; care must be given to when and where it is useful (or not). In the case of multiple selves we locate further challenges. Many highly valued institutions are based on a conception of singular selves; to foster the reality of polyvocality may place such traditions in jeopardy. For example, traditional forms of intimacy are lodged in the capacity to trust—to know the other as he/she truly is. Yet, the polyvocal other may seem little committed; too often he or she may appear glib, superficial, a mere player of games. Similarly, the capacity to hold one responsible depends on a conception of "the one"(or singular agent) who acts. If every voice (action) is only one reflection of a large cast of inner characters, then who is to be blamed or credited for their actions? These are only representative of issues now on the horizon.

From Problems to Prospects

As widely recognized, traditional therapy is based on a medical model of disease and cure. Patients (clients) confront problems—typically indexed as pathologies, adjustment difficulties, dysfunctional relationships, etc.—and it is the task of the therapist to treat the problem in such a way that it is alleviated or removed ("cured"). It is the assumption of "the problem" that underwrites the process of diagnosis and indeed, fuels the development of diagnostic criteria (e.g. the DSM). From a constructionist standpoint, however, this entire array of interlocking presumptions and practices engages in the realist fallacy of presuming that "problems" (diseases) exist independent of our forms of interpretation. For the constructionist the term "problem" is a linguistic integer, and may (or may not) be used to index any condition or state of affairs. It is not the "problems of the world" that determine our ways of talking, for the constructionist, but it is through our linguistic conventions that we determine something to be a problem. Again, this is not to abandon the term or its conventional usages, but rather, to give us pause to consider the consequences. For, as many reason, "problem talk" often reifies a world of anguish; to speak of one's incapacities, an irredeemable other, or a dysfunctional family is to create a world in which one's actions are limited, and very often in which these very limitations sustain the patterns termed problematic.

With these arguments at hand, therapists have developed a new range of practices that attempt to avoid the reification of problems, and shift attention to a discourse of positive prospects. As Riikonen and Smith (1997) put it, "We have been accustomed to talk about analyzing problems as a prerequisite of solving, dissolving or deconstructing them. It seems in most cases more useful to talk about actions, experiences and thoughts which can help to make things better." (p. 25) Most visible in this respect is the work of solution-focused therapies (for example, Berg and deShazer, 1995, deShazer, 1994; O'Hanlon and Weiner-Davis, 1989). The "miracle question" is essentially an invitation to a new domain of dialogue in which the creation of future realities takes precedence over the reification of past problems.

Again, however, it is important to remain sensitive to possible shortcomings in prospect oriented practices. As emphasized in Harlene Anderson's (1997) work, honoring the client reality is essential to a productive relationship. Or as William O'Hanlon (1993) proposes, "if clients don't have a sense that you have heard, acknowledged, and valued them, they will either spend time trying to convince you of the legitimacy of their pain and suffering or they will leave therapy with you." (p. 7) Thus, by rapidly moving toward deconstruction or dissolution of "the problem," the therapist may run the risk of undermining rapport. Further, while it is possible to relativize a client's account of the problem, his/her definition may be importantly tied to relations outside therapy. Regardless of the reconstructive possibilities, for many the "hatred of one's son," "physical abuse," or "incest," will remain problems within the broader culture. To deconstruct such accounts runs the risk of alienating the client from his/her relational surrounds. This point is also related to the earlier discussion of moral engagement. Problems are always such by virtue of a particular tradition of value; to undermine a report of "my problem" is also to place in question the related tradition. None of this is to argue against prospect oriented practices; rather it is to encourage reflection on the use of such practices within the broader matrix of meaning-making.

From Insight to Action

Traditional therapies, linked to the presumption of individual psychological deficit, have also focused on the individual psyche as the site of therapeutic change. Whether, for example, in terms of the transference of psychological energies, catharsis, self-understanding, self-acceptance, re-construal, or cognitive change, most therapeutic practices have been built around the assumption that successful therapy depends primarily on a change in the mind of the individual. Further, it is typically supposed, this change can be accomplished within the therapeutic relationship. The concept of the "therapeutic breakthrough" epitomizes this point of view; once change is accomplished in the therapeutic chamber there is hope that the individual will depart emancipated from the preceding burden with which he/she entered therapy. For discussion purposes let us simply use the phrase "individual insight" to index this class of practices.

Yet, as we shift the emphasis away from individual minds and to discursive relations among individuals, we find the traditional array of practices delimited if not shortsighted. From the constructionist standpoint, the process of generating meaning is continuous, and its form and content likely to shift from one relationship to the next. The individual harbors multiple discursive capacities, and there is no strong reason to anticipate that the meanings generated within the therapeutic relationship will be carried over into outside relationships. The dramatic insight shared between therapist and client is essentially their achievement, a conversational moment that derives its significance from the preceding interchange and cannot easily be lifted out and placed within another conversation remote in time and place.

There is a further and more pro-active shift in therapeutic implications derived from constructionist dialogues. When we locate the source of meaning within dialogic process, we are essentially viewing the meaning-making process as social activity. Meaning, then, is not originated within the mind and stored there for future use, but rather is created in action and regenerated (or not) within subsequent processes of coordination. Following Wittgenstein (1953) we might say that meaning is born of social use. Or, in deShazer's (1994) terms, "Rather than looking behind and beneath the language that clients and therapists use, I think the language they use is all we have to go on...Contrary to the common sense view, change is seen to happen within language: What we talk about and how we talk about it makes a different..." (p. 10).

In this context the primary questions to be asked of therapeutic co-construction are 1) whether a particular form of discourse is actionable outside the therapeutic relationship, and 2) whether the pragmatic consequences of this discourse are desirable. To illustrate, in a Jungian practice one might acquire an entirely specialized vocabulary of individuation, mandalas, the shadow, and so on. Yet, while this vocabulary will enable a fully harmonious relationship to develop within the therapeutic relationship, it is not easily transportable outside. The vocabulary can accomplish little in the way of conversational work. Or, in primal scream therapy one may acquire the capacity for dramatic expressions of rage and anguish. And, while these expressions can produce significant effects in the marketplace of social life, the consequences are not likely to be helpful to the client.

These twin criteria-actionability and pragmatic outcome—have been slow to surface in the constructionist literature and practices. In some degree this relative unconcern is based on the view that therapeutic conversation (along with internal dialogue) yields results in the external world of relationships. Yet, this assumption is largely a promissory note. Much needed are practices specifically dedicated to forging this link. There are good examples extant. For example, White and Murray (1992) and Epston and White have generated a variety of authenticating practices for giving life to newly emerging narratives. They may have celebrations, give prizes with significant people in attendance, or generate "news releases" in which the individual's arrival at a new status is announced to various significant others. White recruits what he terms "The Club of Your Life," which might include anyone, living or dead, actual or imaginary. Epston and his colleagues (Madigan and Epston, 1995) help clients sharing eating disorders to develop politically oriented support groups. Social therapists (Newman and Holzman, 1999; Holzman and Mendez, 2003) encourage and facilitate social activity as a critical component of practice. The emphasis on practical action also helps us to appreciate certain features of some traditional practices. For example, both group and family therapy practices seem favored over individual therapy, as in such contexts one's discourse enters directly into a public arena, and its pragmatic consequences are made more manifest. Further we find new purchase on role-playing therapies. If properly directed, the client gains skills in forms of social doing; otherwise alien forms of expression are incorporated into one's vocabulary of relationship. Buddhist practices of mindfulness and meditation are welcome additions to the vocabulary of action (Kabat Zinn, 2005; Segal, Williams and Teasdale, 2002). In our view, the greatest opportunities for future development lie in this arena of pragmatic consequences of therapeutic conversation.

The Continuing Creation of Practices

As we find, constructionist dialogues invite widespread transformation—both in theory and practice. Not only is the general posture of the therapist toward the client and the therapeutic process displaced significantly, but a range of new and challenging practices has emerged. At the same time, while signs of a broad shift in sensibility are abundant, we continue to confront significant challenges. So far I have treated the contours of change, exploring affinities, practices and challenges. How, then, should we move into the future? Constructionism warns us against freezing our options, or casting any form of therapy in stone. The dialogues of the surrounding culture move on, and if we are to continue effectively to co-create meaning, we must also be prepared for the continuous development of practice.

To facilitate such change, let us return to the contours of the preceding analysis. Specifically, I have developed here eleven dimensions of change—movements from earlier traditions into a world informed by the constructionist dialogues. Yet, these dimensions of change not only allow us to account for recent history; they can also be used to stimulate the kind of reflection necessary for enriching our practices, for moving in yet additional direction. To illustrate, here I have included in the left hand column below each of the constructionist goals, and in the right a therapeutic practice that effectively moves toward this goal:

Flexibility in standpoint	Lynn Hoffman
Consciousness of construction	Milan School
Collaborative orientation	Collaborative Language Systems
Value relevant stance	Feminist therapy
Discursive emphasis	Narrative therapy
Relationship emphasis	"Town" therapy
Polyvocal emphasis	Reflecting team

| Prospect emphasis | Brief/Solution focused |
| Action emphasis | Social therapy |

Now consider the possibility that while a given practice may be highly effective in realizing one constructionist goal, the same practice could be less effective (or even counter productive) in terms of other goals. Not all therapies that emphasize polyvocality, for example, are politically or ideologically engaged; not all practices emphasizing client action are conscious of construction, and so on. Thus, we find that the various goals favored by a constructionist orientation can serve as criteria for reflection. Specifically, given a particular therapeutic practice, we may ask in what ways does it achieve (or not) other desirable goals. More importantly, when it does not achieve one of these goals, can we envision ways in which the practice might be enriched? In effect, by deliberating on the ways in which a given practice does and does not realize certain goals, we enter a creative dialogue from which new practices may emerge.

To illustrate, consider first the now-classic form of narrative therapy outlined by White and Epston (1990). In a constructionist world such a practice would receive high marks for its consciousness of construction, value consciousness, emphasis on relationship, and prospects for action. Yet, as Monk and Gerhart (2003) point out, it differs considerably in its political implications from collaborative practices. A political dimension may be more or less presumed in advance of dialogue. And too, narrative therapy can be resistant to alternative orientations. There is little room within the practice for more traditional standpoints or practices, even if their pragmatic utility might in certain conditions be superior. For example, simply providing positive regard may, in many instances, be just the right resource for the self-punishing client.

Further, there is a strong tendency within narrative therapy to emphasize singularity in story. The attempt is primarily to help the client escape the grasp of a dismal and dominating discourse, and to generate a more useful narrative. Little emphasis is placed either on the multiplicity of stories the client may bring with him/her into therapy or the possibility of moving toward a fluid space of multiple narratives. The productive challenge, then, would be to inquire into ways that the orientation might 1) be rendered more flexible, making use of multiple traditions, and 2) introduce multiple voices and visions into the dialogue. I will expand on this topic in the next chapter.

In a similar manner, we might generate a new wave of solution fo-cused therapies by expanding concern with the political and ideological implications of the therapeutic interchange. For what institutions is a given solution a contribution, for example, and who is suppressed by such a solution. We might also explore new potentials in reflecting team practices when action consequences are placed in focus. What practical consequences follow from various interpretations? Ideologically based therapies might also gain considerably by moving from problem cen-tered discourse ("societal blame") to prospective possibilities. Rather than fighting against societal failings, how can the client participate in creating and working toward a more positive vision? As we find, dra-matic changes in conception and practice of therapy have emerged within the past two decades. However, important challenges are now confronted and the possibilities for new and innovative practices form vistas for an exciting future.

3

Therapeutic Narratives
And Beyond

A man is always a teller of tales, he lives surrounded by his stories and the stories of others, he sees everything that happens to him through them; and he tries to live his life as if he were recounting it.

Jean-Paul Sartre

When people seek psychotherapy they have a story to tell. It is frequently the troubled, bewildered, hurt or angry story of a life or relationship now spoiled. For many it is a story of calamitous events conspiring against their sense of well-being, self-satisfaction, or sense of efficacy. For others the story may concern unseen and mysterious forces insinuating themselves into life's organized sequences, disrupting and destroying. And for still others it is as if, under the illusion of knowing how the world is or ought to be, they have somehow bumped up against trouble for which their favored account has not prepared them. They have discovered an awful reality that now bleeds all past understandings of cogency. Whatever its form, the therapist confronts a narrative—often persuasive and gripping; it is a narrative that may be terminated within a brief period or it may be extended over weeks or months. However, at some juncture the therapist must inevitably respond to this account, and whatever follows within the therapeutic procedure will draw its significance in response to this account.

What options are available to the therapist as he or she now contributes to the unfolding relationship? At least one option is pervasive within the culture, and sometimes used as well within counseling, social work and short-term therapies. It may be viewed as the *advisory option*. For the advisor, the client's story remains relatively inviolate. Its terms of description and forms of explanation remain unchallenged in any significant way. Rather, for the advisor the major attempt is to locate forms of effective action "under the circumstances" as narrated. Thus, for example, if the individual speaks of being depressed because of failure, means are sought for reestablishing efficacy. If the client is rendered ineffectual because of grief, then a program of action may be suggested for overcoming the problem. In effect, the client's life story is accepted as fundamentally accurate for him or her, and the problem is to locate ameliorative forms of action within the story's terms.

There is much to be said on behalf of the advisory option. Within the realm of the relatively ordinary, it is most obviously "reasonable" and most probably effective. Here is the vital stuff of daily coping. Yet, for the more seriously chronic or deeply disturbed client, the advisory option has serious limitations. At the outset, there is little attempt to confront deeper origins of the problem or the complex ways it is sustained. The major concern is in locating a new course of action. Whatever the chain of antecedents, they simply remain the same—often continuing to operate as threats to the future. Further, little attempt is typically made to probe the contours of the story, to determine its relative utility or viability. Could the client be out of social synch, or defining things in a less than optimal way? Such questions often remain unexplored. In accepting "the story as told," the problem definition also remains fixed. As a result the range of possible options for action remains circumscribed. If the problem is said to be failure, for example, the relevant options are geared toward reestablishing success. Other possibilities are thrust to the margins of plausibility. And finally, in the chronic or severe case, the location of action alternatives too often seems superficial. For one who has been frustrated, struggling and desperate for a period of years, for example, simple advice for living may seem little more than whispering in the wind.

In the present chapter two more substantial alternatives to the advisory option will be explored. The first is represented by most traditional forms of psychotherapy and psychoanalytic practice. In its reliance on various assumptions dominant in 20th century science, this orientation may be viewed as modernist. In contrast, much thinking within the postmodern arena—and more specifically postmodern constructionism—forms a powerful challenge to the modernist conception of the narrative. In doing so, new modes of therapeutic procedure are opened.

Therapeutic Narratives in Modernist Context

Much has been written about modernism in the sciences, literature and the arts, and this is scarcely the context for thorough review.[18] However, it is useful to consider briefly a set of pivotal assumptions that have guided activities in the sciences and the allied professions of mental health. For it is this array of assumptions that have largely informed the therapeutic treatment of client narratives. The modernist era in the sciences has been one committed, first of all, to objective and empirically based accounts of what is the case. Whether it be the character of the atom, the gene, or the synapse in the natural sciences, or processes of perception, economic decision making, or organizational development in the social sciences, the major attempt has been to establish bodies of systematic and objective knowledge.

From the modernist standpoint, empirical knowledge is communicated through scientific languages. Narratives are essentially structures of language, and insofar as narratives are generated within the scientific milieu they can, on the modernist account, function as conveyors of the truth. Thus, the narratives of the novelist are labeled as "fiction," and are considered irrelevant to serious scientific pursuits. People's narratives of their lives, what has happened to them and why, are not necessarily fictions. But, as the behavioral scientist proclaims, they are notoriously inaccurate and unreliable. Thus, they are considered of limited value in understanding the individual's life, and far less preferable than the empirically based accounts of the trained scientist. As a result, the narrative accounts of the scientist are accorded the highest credibility, and are set above and apart from the homespun stories of everyday life and the markets of public entertainment.

The mental health profession today is largely an outgrowth of modernist beliefs and shares deeply in its assumptions. Thus from Freud to contemporary cognitive therapists, the general belief is that the professional therapist functions (or ideally should function) as a scientist. By virtue of such activities as scientific training, research experience, knowledge of the scientific literature, and countless hours of systematic observation and thought within the therapeutic situation, the professional is armed with knowledge. To be sure, contemporary knowledge is incomplete, and more research is ever required. But the knowledge of the contemporary professional is far superior to that of the turn-of-the-century therapist, so it is said, and the future can only bring further improvements. Thus, with few exceptions, therapeutic theories (whether behavioral, systemic, psychodynamic, or experiential/humanist) contain explicit assumptions regarding a) the underlying cause or basis of pathology, b) the location of this cause within the client or his/her relationships, c) the means by which such problems can be diagnosed, and d) the means by which the pathology may be eliminated. In effect, the trained professional enters the therapeutic arena with a well developed narrative for which there is abundant support within the community of scientific peers.

It is this background that establishes the therapist's posture toward the client's narrative. For the client's narrative is, after all, made of the flimsy stuff of daily stories—replete with whimsy, metaphor, wishful thinking, and distorted memories. The scientific narrative, by contrast, has the seal of professional approval. From this vantage point we see that the therapeutic process must inevitably result in the slow but inevitable replacement of the client's story with the therapist's. The client's story does not remain a free-standing reflection of truth, but rather, as questions are asked and answered, descriptions and explanations are reframed, and affirmation and doubt are disseminated by the therapist, the client's narrative is either destroyed or incorporated—but in any case replaced—by the professional account. The client's account is transformed by the psychoanalyst into a tale of family romance, by the Rogerian into a struggle against conditional regard, and so on. It is this process of replacing the client's story with the professional that is so deftly described in Donald Spence's <u>Narrative Truth and Historical Truth</u>. As Spence surmises,

> *(The therapist) is constantly making decisions about the form and status of the patient's material. Specific listening conventions...help to guide these decisions. If, for example, the analyst assumes that contiguity indicates causality, then he will hear a sequence of disconnected statements as a causal chain; at some later time, he might make an interpretation that would make this assumption explicit. If he assumes that transference predominates and that the patient is always talking, in more or less disguised fashion, about the analyst, then he will "hear" the material in that way and make some kind of ongoing evaluation of the state of the transference.* (p. 129)

Such replacement procedures do have certain therapeutic advantages. For one, as the client gains "real insight" into his/her problems, the problematic narrative is thereby removed. The client is thus furnished with an alternative reality that holds promise for future well-being. In effect, the failure story with which the client entered therapy is swapped for an invitation to a success story. And, similar to the advisory option outlined earlier, the new story is likely to suggest alternative lines of action—forming or dissolving relationships, operating under a daily regimen, submitting to therapeutic procedures, and so on. Within the professional story there are new and more hopeful, things to do. And too, by providing the client a scientific formulation, the therapist has played his/her appointed role in the family of cultural rituals in which the ignorant, the failing, and the weak seek counsel from the wise, superior, and strong. It is indeed a comforting ritual to all who will submit.

Yet, in spite of these advantages, there is substantial reason for concern. I shall not treat here the many ideological and conceptual critiques of modernist therapy accumulated over recent decades. And the case against the modernist objectification of mental disorder was amply addressed in the preceding chapter. Over and above these problems, there are specific shortcomings in the modernist orientation to client narrative. There is, for one, a substantial imperious thrust to the modernist approach. Not only is the therapist's narrative never placed under threat, but the therapeutic procedure virtually ensures that it will win out. In Spence's terms, "the search space (within therapeutic interaction) can be infinitely expanded until the (therapist's) answer is discovered and...there is no possibility of finding a negative solution, of deciding that the (therapist's) search has failed." (p. 108) Thus, regardless of the complexity, sophistication or value of the client's account, it is eventually replaced by a narrative created before his/her entry into therapy and the contours over which he/she has no control.

It is not simply that therapists from a given school will ensure their clients come away bearing beliefs in their particular account. By virtue of their parochial commitments, the ultimate aim of most traditional schools of therapy is hegemonic. All other schools of thought, and their associated narratives, should succumb. In general psychoanalysts wish to eradicate behavior modification; cognitive-behavioral therapists see psychoanalysis as misguided; systems therapists find cognitive therapists myopic, and so on. Yet, the most immediate and potentially injurious consequences are reserved for the client. For in the end, the structure of the procedure furnishes the client a lesson in inferiority. The client is indirectly informed that he/she is ignorant, insensitive, or emotionally incapable of comprehending what has taken place and why. In contrast, the therapist is positioned as the all knowing and wise—a model to which the client might aspire. The situation is all the more lamentable owing to the fact that in occupying the superior role, the therapist fails to reveal its weaknesses. Almost nowhere are the wobbly foundations of the therapist's account made known; almost nowhere do the therapist's personal doubts, foibles, and failings come to light. And the client is thus confronted with a vision of human perfection that is as unattainable as the heroism of Hollywood film.

The modernist orientation suffers as well from the fixedness of the narrative formulations. As we have seen, modernist approaches to therapy begin with an a priori narrative, justified by claims to a scientific base. Because it is sanctioned as scientific, this narrative is relatively closed to alteration. Minor modifications may be entertained, but the system itself bears the weight of established doctrine. To the extent that such narratives become the client's reality, and his/her actions are guided accordingly, life options for the client are severely delimited. Of all possible modes of acting in the world, one is set on a course emphasizing ego autonomy, self-actualization, rational appraisal, emotional expressiveness, and so on depending on the particular brand of therapy selected. Or to put it otherwise, each form of modernist therapy carries with it an image of the "fully functioning" or "good" individual; like a fashion plate, this image serves as the guiding model for the therapeutic outcome.

This constriction of life possibilities is all the more problematic because the guiding image is decontextualized. That is, the therapist's narrative is an abstract formalization—cut away from particular cultural and historical circumstances. None of the modernist narratives deal with the specific conditions of living in ghetto poverty, with a brother who has AIDs, with a child who has Down 's syndrome, with an attractive boss who is sexually solicitous, and so on. In contrast to the complex details that crowd the corners of daily life—which are indeed life itself—modernist narratives are non-specific. They aspire toward universality, and on this account, often say very little about particularistic circumstance. As a result these narratives may be precariously insinuated into the life circumstances of the individual. In this sense, they can be clumsy and insensitive, failing to register the particularities of the circumstances. To emphasize self-fulfillment to a woman living in a household with three small children and a mother-in-law with Alzheimer's is not likely to be beneficial. To press a Park Avenue attorney for increased emotional expressiveness in his daily routines is of doubtful assistance. To pump up the self-regard of an individual whose spouse is a drug addict may be beside the point.[19]

Therapeutic Realities in Postmodern Context

As described in the opening chapters, the arguments leading toward social construction form a major challenge to the modernist view of knowledge and science. In an important sense, constructionism is a child of the "postmodern turn" in cultural life.[20] In the present context, constructionist arguments undermine claims to scientific truth, whether offered by natural scientists or therapeutic practitioners. Or to extend the case, narrative accounts are not replicas of reality but the devices from which reality is constructed. To be sure, as in the natural sciences, some may be found more truthful or objective than others, but this is owing to the local conventions of language use. Truth may be achieved parochially, but not transcendentally.

Such arguments form a major challenge to the modernist orientation to therapy. At the outset they remove the factual justification of the modernist narratives of pathology and cure. They undermine the unquestioned status of the therapist as scientific authority, with privileged knowledge of cause and cure. The therapist's narratives thus take their place along side the myriad possibilities available in the culture, not transcendentally superior, but differ in pragmatic implications. By the same token significant questions must be raised with the traditional practice of replacing the client's stories with the fixed and narrow alternatives of the modernist therapist. There is no justification outside the small community of like-minded therapists for hammering the client's complex and richly detailed life into a single, pre-formulated narrative, a narrative that may be of little relevance or promise for the client's subsequent life conditions. And finally, there is no broad justification for the traditional status hierarchy that both demeans and frustrates the client. The therapist and client form a community to which both bring resources and from which the contours of the future may be carved.

The Pragmatics of Narration

Narrative accounts in modernist frame serve as potential representations of reality—true or false in their capacity to represent "what actually happened." Thus, in the therapeutic case, if the narrative reflects a recurring pattern of maladaptive action, one begins to explore alternative ways of behaving. Or, if it indicates the onset of pathology, drugs can be prescribed. Within the modernist view, the therapist's narrative has a privileged status in prescribing an optimal way of life. In contrast, for most therapists informed by the perspectivalism of the postmodern era, the modernist concern with narrative accuracy ceases to compel. Narrative truth cannot ultimately be distinguished from historical truth, except from within the confines of a particular tradition. What, then, is the function of narrative reconstruction?

Most existing accounts now point to the potential of such reconstructions to reorient the individual, to open new courses of action that are more fulfilling and more adequately suited to the individual's capacities and proclivities. Thus, the client may alter or dispose of earlier narratives, not because they are inaccurate, but because they are dysfunctional in his/her particular circumstances.

Yet, the question must be raised, in precisely what way(s) is a narrative "useful." How does a language of self-understanding guide, direct or inform lines of action? What does the story do for (or to) the client? Two answers to this question pervade post-empiricist camps at present, and both are importantly flawed. On the one side is the metaphor of language as a lens. On this account, a narrative construction is a vehicle through which the world is seen. It is through the lens of narrative that the individual identifies objects, persons, actions, and so on. As many argue, it is on the basis of the world as seen, and not on the world as it is, that the individual determines a course of action. Thus, one who sees their life as a tragic fall, would perceive life's unfolding events in these terms. Yet, to take this position is to view the individual as isolated and solipsistic—simply stewing in the juices of his/her own constructions. The possibilities for survival are minimal, for there is no means of escaping encapsulation in the internal system of construals. Further, such an account buys a range of notorious epistemological problems. How, for example, does the individual develop the lens? From whence the first construction? For if there is no world outside that which is internally constructed, there would be no means of understanding, and thus of developing or fashioning the lens. How can we defend the view that the sounds and markings employed in human interchange are somehow transported into the mind to impose order on the perceptual world? This was indeed Benjamin Lee Whorf's proposal, but it is a view that never succeeded in being more than controversial. The argument for language as lens seems poorly taken.

The major alternative to this view holds that narrative constructions are internal models, forms of story that can be interrogated by the individual as guides to action. Again, there is no brief made for the truth of the model; the narrative operates simply as an enduring structure that informs and directs action. Thus, for example, a person who features himself as a hero whose feats of bravery and intelligence will prevail against all odds, finds life unworkable. Through therapy he realizes that such a view not only places him in impossible circumstances but works against close feelings of intimacy and interdependence with his wife and children. A new story is worked out in which the individual comes to see himself as a champion not for himself, but for his family. His heroism will be achieved through their feelings of happiness, and will thus depend importantly on their assessments of his actions. It is this transformed image that is to guide subsequent actions. While there is a certain wisdom to this position, it is again problematic. Stories of this variety are in themselves both idealized and abstract. As such they can seldom dictate behavior in complex, ongoing interaction. What does the new story of self say, for example, about the best reaction to his wife's desires for him to spend fewer hours at work and more with the family, or how should he respond to a new job offer, challenging and profitable, but replete with risk? Stories as internal models are not only bare of specific directives or implications, but they remain static. The individual moves through numerous situations and relationships—a parent dies, his son is tempted by drugs, an attractive neighbor acts seductively, and so on. Yet, the narrative model remains inflexible—unbending and of obscure relevance. The "model in the head" is largely useless.

Yet, there is a third way of understanding narrative utility, one that grows out of the constructionist emphasis on the pragmatics of language. Here it is proposed that narratives gain their utility primarily within social interchange. They are significant entries into ongoing relationships—essential for maintaining the intelligibility and coherence of social life, useful in drawing people together, creating distance, and so on. Stories of the self enable public identities to be established, the past rendered acceptable, and the rituals of relationship to unfold with ease. The utility of these stories derives from their success as moves within these relational arenas—in terms of their adequacy as reactions to previous moves, or as instigators to what follows.

Consider, for example, a story of failure—how one tried one's best to pass a professional exam but failed. As we have seen, the story is neither true nor false in itself; it is simply one construction of events among many. However, as this story is inserted into various forms of relationship—into the games or dances of the culture—its effects are strikingly varied. If a friend has just related a story of great personal achievement, one's story of failure is likely to act as a repressive force, and alienate the friend who otherwise anticipated a congratulatory reaction. If, in contrast, the friend had just revealed a personal failure, to share one's own failings is likely to be reassuring and to solidify the friendship. Similarly, to relate one's story of failure to one's mother may elicit a warm and sympathetic reaction—in effect, enabling her to be a "mother;" but to share it with a wife who worries each month over making ends meet may produce both frustration and anger.

To put it otherwise, a story is not simply a story. It is itself a situated action, a performance that affects the course of social life. It acts so as to create, sustain or alter worlds of social relationship. In these terms, it is insufficient that the client and therapist negotiate a new form of self-understanding that seems realistic, aesthetic, and uplifting within the dyad. It is not the dance of meaning within the therapeutic context that is primarily at stake. Rather, the significant question is whether the new shape of meaning is serviceable within the social arena outside these confines. How, for example, does the story of oneself as "hero of the family group" play for a wife who dislikes her dependent status, a boss who is a "self-made woman," or a rebellious son? What forms of action does the story invite in each of these situations; what kinds of dances are engendered, facilitated or sustained as a result? It is evaluation at this level that seems most crucial for the joint consideration of therapist and client.

Transcending Narrative

The focus on narrative pragmatics sets the stage for perhaps the most important argument of the chapter. As noted earlier, for many therapists making the postmodern turn in therapy, the narrative continues to be viewed as a condition of mind, either a form of internal lens through which life is seen, or an internal model for the guidance of action. In light of the preceding discussion of pragmatics, these conceptions are found lacking in three important respects. First, each retains the individualist cast of modernism, in that the final resting place of the narrative construction is within the mind of the single individual. As we have reconsidered the utility of the narrative, we have moved outward—from the individual's mind to the relationships constituted by the narrative in action. Narratives exist in the telling, and tellings are constituents of relational forms—for good or ill. Second, the metaphors of the lens and the internal model both favor singularity in narrative. That is, both tend to presume the functionality of a single formulation of self-understanding. The individual possesses "a lens" for comprehending the world, it is said, not a repository of lenses; and through therapy one comes to possess "a new narrative truth," it is often put, not a multiplicity of truths. From the pragmatic standpoint, the presumption of singularity operates against functional adequacy. Each narrative of the self may function well in certain circumstances, but lead to miserable outcomes in others. To have only a single means of making self intelligible, then, is to limit the range of relationships or situations in which one can function satisfactorily. For example, to carry a narrative of righteous indignation—how one was unjustly treated by the world—may be useful with sympathetic friends. Bonds of friendship can even be strengthened through such a telling. However, in conversations with one's boss or with one's children, the narrative may provoke or estrange. To be over-skilled or over-prepared in telling this will vastly reduce one's potentials. From the present perspective, narrative multiplicity is vastly to be preferred.

Finally, the psychological conception of narrative favors belief in or commitment to one's story. Such a conception suggests that the individual lives within the narrative as a system of understanding. One "sees the world in this way," as it is said, and the narrative is thus "true for the individual." Or the transformed story of self is "the new reality;" it constitutes a "new belief about self" to support and sustain the individual. Again, however, as we consider the social utility of narrative, traditions of belief and commitment become suspect. To be committed to a given story of self, to adopt it as "true for me," is to vastly limit one's possibilities of relating. To believe that one is successful is thus as debilitating in certain respects as believing that one is a failure. Both are only stories after all, and each may bear fruit within a particular range of contexts and relationships. To crawl inside one and make a home is to forego the other, and thus to reduce the range of contexts and relationships in which one is adequate. One is less flexible in moving within the relational flow.

To frame the issue in another way, postmodern consciousness favors a thoroughgoing relativism in expressions of identity. On the meta-theoretical level it invites a multiplicity of accounts of reality, while recognizing the historically and culturally situated contingency of each. There are only accounts of truth within differing conversations, and no conversation is transcendentally privileged. Thus, for the postmodern practitioner a multiplicity of self-accounts is invited, but a commitment to none. From this standpoint the client should be encouraged, on the one hand, to explore a variety of narrative formulations, but discouraged from commitment to any particular "truth of self." The narrative constructions thus remain fluid, open to the shifting tides of circumstance—to the forms of dance that provide fullest sustenance.

Can such a conclusion be tolerated? Is the individual thus reduced to a social con artist, adopting whatever posture of identity that garners the highest payoff? Certainly the constructionist emphasis is on flexibility in self-identification, but this does not simultaneously imply that the individual is either duplicitous or scheming. To speak of duplicity is to presume that there is a "true telling" that is otherwise available. Such a view is deeply problematic and thus abandoned. One may interpret one's actions as duplicitous or sincere, but these ascriptions are, after all, simply components of different stories. Similarly, to presume that the individual possesses private motives, including a rational calculus of self-presentation (the psychological basis of a "con") is again to sustain the modernist view of the self-contained individual. From the constructionist standpoint the relationship takes priority over the individual self. That is, selves are only realized as a byproduct of relatedness. Thus, to shift in the form and content of self narration from one relationship to another is neither deceitful nor self-serving in the traditional sense. Rather, it is to honor the various modes of relationship in which one is enmeshed. It is to take seriously the multiple and varied forms of human connectedness that make up a life. Adequate and fulfilling actions are only so in the terms of criteria generated within the various forms of relationship themselves.[21]

Therapeutic Moves

As we find, therapy as a means toward narrative reconstruction or replacement does not fully realize either the full implications of constructionist theory or to facilitate the full possibilities for human functioning. From a thoroughgoing constructionism, the emphasis is placed on narrative within the broader social process of generating meaning. This involves an appreciation of the contextual relativity of meaning, an acceptance of indeterminacy, the generative exploration of a multiplicity of meanings, and the understanding that there is no necessity for adhering to an invariant story or searching for a definitive identity. The continuous challenge is that of moving adequately within the relational flow. "Re-authoring" or "re-storying" seems then, but a first-order therapeutic approach, one which implies the replacement of a dysfunctional master narrative with a more functional one. At the same time this result carries the seeds of a prescriptive rigidity—one which might also serve to confirm an illusion that it is possible to develop a set of principles or codes which can be invariantly applied irrespective of relational context.

From a certain standpoint, one may also venture that this very rigidity is constitutive of the difficulties which people often bring to the therapeutic situation. This possibility is worthy of attention. Just as psychotherapists may be restrained by a limiting code, so people who describe their lives as problematic often seem trapped within a limiting vocabulary, behavioral codes and constitutive conventions from which the contours of their lives are molded. Acting in terms of a singular narrative and its associated actions, one is not only restrained from exploring alternative possibilities but can become imprisoned in painful transactional patterns with those about them.

If language provides the matrix for all human understanding, then psychotherapy may be aptly construed as "linguistic activity in which conversation about a problem generates the development of new meanings" (Goolishian and Winderman, 1988, p. 139). Put differently, psychotherapy may be thought of as a process of semiosis—the forging of meaning in the context of collaborative discourse. It is a process through which the meaning of events is transformed via a fusion of the horizons of the participants, alternative ways of narrating events are developed, and new stances toward self and others evolve. A crucial component of this process may inhere not only in the alternative ways of accounting generated by the discourse but also in the different order of meaning which concurrently emerges.

To help another achieve the perspective that comes from seeing that we cannot see implies first a release from the tyranny of the implied authority of governing beliefs. Given the linguistic constitution of our world models, required is a transformative dialogue in which new understandings are negotiated together with a new set of premises about meaning. Further, we must nourish an expectant attitude toward the as yet unseen, the as yet unstoried, the "meaning ahead of the text" (Ricouer, 1971). In terms of Bateson's (1972) distinctions between levels of learning, it is a move beyond learning to replace one punctuation of a situation with another (Level 1), to learning new modes of punctuation (Level 2), to evolving what Keeney (1983, p. 159) calls "a change of the premises underlying an entire system of punctuation habits." (Level 3) It is a progression from learning new meanings to developing new categories of meaning, to ultimately transforming ones premises about the nature of meaning itself.

For any of these transformations to occur, a context needs to be established which facilitates their emergence. At the outset there is much to be said for Goolishian and Anderson's (1991) emphasis on creating a climate where clients have the experience of being heard, of having both their point of view and feelings understood, of feeling themselves confirmed and accepted. Invited are endeavors to understand the client's point of view, to convey an understanding of how it makes sense to the person given the premises from which the viewpoint arises. At the same time this does not imply a necessary commitment to the client's premises. Rather, it serves as a contextual validation for a particular account, a validation that is enables client and therapist to reconstitute this reality as a conversational object—now vulnerable to a new infusion of meaning. How is this process to proceed? There is no single answer to this question, just as there can be no principled constraint over the number of possible conversations. However, therapists sensitive to the postmodern dialogues have been highly creative in developing conceptually congenial practices. Hoffman (1990) sets the contours for "an art of lenses." Goolishian and Anderson (1992) employ a form of interested inquiry, asking questions that simultaneously credit the client's reality while pressing it toward evolution. Andersen and his colleagues (1991) have developed the practice of the reflecting team, individuals who observe the therapeutic encounter and then share their opinions with both therapist and client. In this way, the aura of single authority (the therapist) is reduced, an appreciation for multiple realities is generated, and the client is furnished with a variety of resources for proceeding. White and Epston (1990) employ letters (and other written documents) to help clients to re-author their lives. Letters may be written by both clients and the therapist. Penn (2001) also relies on client letter-writing, but with the major emphasis on generating a dialogic process within the clients' stories, so that new openings are subsequently forged for conversations with others. Hanlon and Wilk (1987) lay out an array of conversational means by which client-therapist negotiation may proceed toward a dissolution of the putative problem. DeShazer (1991) encourages conversation on solutions (as opposed to problems), and Friedman and Fanger (1991) on positive possibilities. Lipchik (1993) emphasizes client talk about balancing the various goods and bads in exiting alternatives, to replace an either/or orientation with a both/and. Many therapists place a strong emphasis on positive construction of self and life circumstances (see for example Durrant and Kowalski, 1993). Fruggeri (1992) encourages different descriptions of given events, new ways of connecting behaviors and events, and a process of continuous reflexivity. Amorim and Cavalcante (1992) help disabled adolescents to produce puppet shows in which they narrate their life conditions and possibilities.

Yet, simply because these therapeutic forms grow from the soil of a postmodern constructionism, does not mean that all other therapies are outmoded or abandoned. On the contrary, as outlined in preceding chapters, a constructionist standpoint—unlike its meta-theoretical predecessors—does not attempt to eradicate alternative languages of understanding and their associated practices. Such prefixes as "is true," "is objective," "is more successful in producing cures," may be removed from discussions of the alternatives. However, all theories of therapy, all forms of therapeutic practice, must be considered in terms of what they add (or subtract) from the conversational matrix we call therapy. Couches, dream analyses, positive regard, strategic interventions, circular questioning, are all entries into the broader vocabulary of the profession. They invite certain lines of interchange and action, and suppress others.

By the same token, we must view the modernist attempt to replace lay languages (of "ignorance") with scientific languages—and typically a univocal language of the true—as unnecessarily and detrimentally constraining. The common languages by which people live their daily lives have enormous pragmatic potential. Living room languages, street languages, spiritual languages, new age languages—these and others are prime movers in the culture. To restrict their entry into the therapeutic setting is to reduce the possibilities for conversation. Belief is not in question here, for the concept of belief (as indexing a mental state) is itself deeply suspect. Rather, the major challenge concerns the potential of the therapeutic conversation to alter the course of events.

More generally, we may ask whether our languages and practices can liberate participants from static and delimiting conventions of understanding and enable a full flexibility of relationship. Can those turning to the therapist in times of trouble come to transcend the restraints imposed by their erstwhile reliance on a determinate set of meanings and be freed from the struggle than ensues from imposing their beliefs on self and others? Hopefully for some, new solutions to problems can become apparent, while for others a richer set of narrative meanings will emerge. For still others a stance toward meaning itself can perhaps evolve; one which betokens that tolerance of uncertainty, that freeing of self which comes from acceptance of unbounded relativity of meaning. For those who adopt it, this stance offers the prospect of a creative participation in the unending and unfolding meaning of life.

> *I will try*
> *to fasten into order enlarging grasps of disorder, widening*
> *scope, but enjoying the freedom that*
> *Scope eludes my grasp, that there is no finality of vision,*
> *that I have perceived nothing completely,*
> *that tomorrow a new walk is a new walk.*
>
> A.R. Ammons, Carson's Inlet

Part II

Mental Health
As Oppression

4

Deficit Discourse
And Cultural Enfeeblement

... we multiply distinctions, then
Deem that our puny boundaries are things
That we perceive, and not that which we have made.

William Wordsworth

Judging from my many colleagues, students and friends engaged in therapeutic practices, I believe they generally share a strong and genuine commitment to a vision of human betterment. Further, although research on
therapeutic efficacy is inevitably equivocal, it is clear that many who seek
help believe their condition is improved as a result. Yet, my concern in the
present offering is with the paradoxical consequences of the prevailing
vision of human betterment, and the pervasive hope that these professions can improve the quality of cultural life. For there is reason to believe that in certain important respects, present efforts to alleviate human
suffering simultaneously contribute to its expansion. The problem lies
primarily within the prevailing construction of human deficit. In its discourses of deficit—of disease, pathology, and dysfunction—the mental
health professions prosper through the expansion of human misery. This
is not a trivial accusation, and there are more positive options open to us.
In the present chapter I focus on the impact of deficit discourse; in the
subsequent chapter attention will turn to the related issues of biologizing
human problems and pharmacological treatment. Some background is
useful in exploring the construction of mental illness.

Psychological Discourse: Pictorial or Pragmatic?

In order to appreciate the nature and magnitude of the problem, it is useful to consider the relation between the language we use in describing or explaining the mind, and its referents, namely the workings of the mind itself. Here a crucial distinction can be drawn between two views of such language. Most commonly we employ such terms as "thinking," "feeling," "hoping," "fearing," and the like *pictorially*. That is, in the same way we use different names in referring to individual persons, or different words to talk about various objects around us (e.g. trees, houses, dogs, cars), we use mental terms as if they reflected distinct conditions of mind. The statement, "I am angry," is intended, by common convention, to describe a state of mind, differing from other states such as joy, embarrassment, or ecstasy.

The vast majority of therapeutic specialists also proceed in the same manner. Therapists listen for hours to their clients to ascertain the quality and character of their "inner life"—their thoughts, emotions, unarticulated fears, conflicts, repressions, and most focally, "the world as they experience it." As commonly presumed, the individual's language provides a vehicle for "inner access"—revealing or setting forth to the professional the character of the not-directly-observed. And, as it is further reasoned, this task is essential to the therapeutic outcome—whether for reasons of furnishing the therapist with helpful information about the client's mental condition, or for promoting client self-insight, enhancing self-esteem, inducing catharsis, reducing guilt and so on.

Yet, while we commonly employ psychological language as if it describes or pictures the internal world, such an assumption is deeply flawed. Consider some of the problems attendant upon attaching psychological terms—"attitudes," "anxiety," "intentions," "feelings" and the like to specific conditions in the mind:

- At the outset, how could consciousness turn in upon itself to identify its own states? How can experience become an object to itself? Can a mirror reflect its own image?

- What are the characteristics of mental states by which we can identify them? By what criteria do we distinguish, let us say, among states of anger, fear and love? What is the color of hope, the size of a thought, or the shape of anger? Why do none of these attributes seem quite applicable to mental states? Is it because our observations of the states prove to us that they are not? What would we be observing in this case?

- Could we identify our mental states through their physiological manifestations—blood pressure, heart rate, etc. Do I know I am thinking by checking my blood pressure, or that I have hope by feeling my neurological activity? And, if we were sufficiently sensitive to differing physiological conditions, how would we know to which states each referred? Does increased pulse rate indicate anger more than love, or hope more than despair?

- How can we be certain when we identify such states correctly? Could other processes (e.g. repression, defense) not prevent accurate self-appraisal? (Perhaps anger is eros after all.)

- By what criterion could we judge that what we experience as "certain recognition" of a mental state is indeed certain recognition? Wouldn't this recognition ("I am certain in my assessment.") require yet another round of self-assessments ("I am certain that what I am experiencing is certainty..."), the results of which would require additional processes of internal identification, and so on in an infinite regress?

- Although we may all agree in our use of mental terms (that we experience fear, ecstasy, or joy, for example on particular occasions) how do we know that our own subjective experiences resemble those of others? By what process could we possibly determine whether my "fear" is equivalent to yours? How then do I know I possess what everyone else calls "fear"?

- How are we to account for the disappearance from the culture of many mental terms popular in previous centuries, along with the passing fashions in mental terminology of the present century? (Whatever happened to melancholy, sublimity, neuralgia, and the inferiority complex?) Have the words disappeared because such processes no longer exist in mortal minds?

- How are we to account for the substantial variations in psychological vocabulary from one culture to another? Did we once have the same mental events as the primitive tribesman, for example the emotion of "fago," described by Lutz (1989) in her studies of the Ifaluk? Have we lost the capacity to experience this emotion? Is it lurking somewhere within the core of our being, buried beneath the layers of Western sophistication? By what standards could we decide one way or another?

These problems have long resisted solution, and strongly suggest that using mental language in pictorial fashion is deeply misleading. Moreover such language functions to objectify the mental world, that is, to create its referents as objectively real. In this way such language engages in a *fallacy of misplaced concreteness*. We treat as concrete the objects of the discourse rather than the discourse itself. This is not to say that "nothing is going on" within the individual when he/she is shouting in anger, is locked in an embrace, or hears ominous sounds in the dark. However, there is nothing about these human conditions that demands a distinctly mental vocabulary, any more than a vocabulary of physiology or atomic physics. To use mental language pictorially is to create the Western world of the mind as universal—with thought, emotion, and illness true for all people.

Let us contrast the pictorial orientation to mental language with yet another, one we may term pragmatic. For this purpose, let us bracket the view of mental language as a mirror of inner states, and consider such language as feature of social relationships. That is, we may venture that psychological language obtains its meaning and significance primarily from the way in which it is used in human interaction. Thus, when I say "I am unhappy" about a given state of affairs, the term "unhappy" is not rendered meaningful or appropriate according to its relationship to the state of my neurons or my phenomenological field. Rather, the report plays a significant social function. It may be used, for example, to call an end to a set of deteriorating conditions, enlist support and/or encouragement, or to invite further opinion. Both the conditions of the report and the functions it can serve are also circumscribed by social convention. The phrase, "I am deeply sad" can be satisfactorily reported at the death of a close relative but not the demise of a spring moth. A report of depression can secure others' concern and support; however it cannot easily function as a greeting, an invitation to laughter, or a commendation. In this sense to use mental language is more like having a warm smile or an embrace than a mirror of the interior, more like a strong grip between trapeze artists than a map of inner conditions. In effect, mental terms are used by people in carrying out relationships.[22]

Cultural Consequences of Deficit Discourse

The pervasive stance toward psychological discourse in Western culture is decidedly pictorial. We generally accept persons' accounts of their subjective states as valid (at least for them). If sophisticated, we may wonder if they are fully aware of their feelings, or have been misled in an attempt to protect themselves from what is "really" there. And, if scientific in bent, we may wish to know the distribution of various mental states (e.g. loneliness, depression) in the society more generally, the conditions under which they occur (e.g. stress, burnout), and the means for their alteration (e.g. the comparative efficacy of differing therapies). However, we are unlikely to question the existence of the reality to which such terms seem to refer; and because the prevailing conception of mental life remains generally unchallenged, we seldom inquire into the utility or desirability of such terms in daily life. If the language exists because the mental states exist, there is little reason for critical appraisal of the language. By common standards, to disapprove of the language of the mind is tantamount to finding the shape of the earth disagreeable.

Yet, if we view psychological discourse from a pragmatic perspective, mental language loses its function as "truth bearing." One cannot claim rights to language use on grounds that existing terms "name what there is." Further, significant questions are invited concerning the existing terminologies. For, in effect, the "ways we talk" are intimately intertwined with patterns of cultural life. They sustain and support certain ways of doing things, and prevent others from emerging. From the pragmatic perspective it is of paramount important, then, to inquire into the effects on human relationships of the prevailing vocabularies of the mind. Given our goals for human betterment, do these vocabularies facilitate or obstruct? And, most important for present purposes, what kinds of social patterns are facilitated (or prevented) by the existing vocabulary of psychological deficit? How do the terms of the mental health professions, terms such as "neurosis," "cognitive dysfunction," "depression," "post-traumatic stress disorder," "character disorder," "repression," "narcissism" and so on, function within the culture more generally? Do such terms lend themselves to desirable forms of human relationship, should the vocabulary be expanded, and are there more promising alternatives? There are no simple answers to such questions; neither is there an active discussion. My purpose here is not so much to develop a final answer as to generate a forum for challenging dialogue.

Grounds for such discussion have been laid in several relevant arenas. In a range of highly critical volumes Thomas Szasz (1961; 1963; 1970) has argued that concepts of mental illness are not demanded by observation. Rather, he proposes they function much as social myths, and are used (or misused, from his perspective) largely as means of social control. Sarbin and Mancuso (1980) echo these arguments in their focus on the concept of schizophrenia as a social construction. Similarly, Ingelby (1980) has demonstrated the ways in which categories of mental illness are negotiated so as to serve the values or ideological investments of the profession. Kovel (1980) proposes that the mental health professions are essentially forms of industry that operate largely in the service of existing economic structures. Feminist thinkers have explored the ways in which nosologies of illness, diagnosis and treatment are all biased against women and favor the continuation of the patriarchy (Brodsky and Hare-Mustin, 1980; Hare-Mustin and Marecek, 1988). And drawing from Foucault's (1978, 1979) analysis of knowledge-power relationships, Rose (1985), and Schacht (1985) have examined various ways in which mental testing, and the realities which it creates, serve the controlling interests of the culture. All of these critics question, then, the truth bearing capacity of mental language, and pinpoint oppressive consequences of current language usage.[23]

There is much to be said about the ways in which mental deficit language functions within the culture, and not all of it is critical. On the positive side, for example, the vocabulary of the mental health professions does serve to render the alien familiar, and thus less fearsome. Rather than viewing unusual behavior as "the work of the devil" or "frighteningly strange," for example, we have standardized labels, signifying that indeed, such behavior is not uncommon, of long familiarity to the sciences. At the same time, this process of familiarization invites one to replace repugnance and fear with more humane reactions—sympathetic reactions of the kind appropriate to the physically ill. One can be more nurturing and understanding to someone suffering from a "disease" than one who seems intentionally obstructive. Further, because the mental health professions are allied with science, and science is socially represented as a progressive or problem solving activity, scientific labeling also invites a hopeful attitude toward the future. One need not be burdened with the belief that today's illnesses are forever.

For most of us current discursive practices represent distinct improvements over many early predecessors (See Rosen, 1968). Yet, optimism on such matters is hardly merited. For there is a substantial "down side" to existing intelligibilities, and as I shall hope to demonstrate, these problems are of continuously increasing magnitude. Consider, in particular, the functioning of mental deficit vocabularies in engendering and facilitating forms of what might be viewed as cultural enfeeblement:

Social Hierarchy

How may I fault thee? Let me count the ways...

Impulsive personality	Low self-esteem
Malingering	Narcissism
Reactive depression	Bulimia
Anorexia	Neurasthenia
Mania	Hypochondriasis
Attention deficit disorder	Dependent personality
Psychopathia	Frigidity
External control orientation	Authoritarianism
Anti-social personality	Transvestism
Exhibtionism	Agoraphobia
Seasonal affective Disorder...	Social anxiety

Although often boasting a position of scientific neutrality, it has long been recognized that the helping professions are inevitably premised on assumptions of the cultural good (Hartmann, 1960; Masserman, 1960). Professional visions of "healthy functioning" are suffused with cultural ideals of personhood (London, 1986; Margolis, 1966) and associated political ideologies (Leifer, 1990). In this context we find, then, that mental deficit terms operate as evaluative devices, demarking the position of individuals along culturally implicit dimensions of good and bad. We may often feel a degree of sympathy for the person who complains of incapacitating depression, anxiety, or a Type-A personality. However, such sympathies are often tinged with a sense of self-satisfaction, for the complaint simultaneously casts one into a position of superiority. In each case the other is marked by failure—insufficient buoyancy, level headedness, calm, control, and so on. All of the above terms, for example, are discrediting; all point to a form of inferiority.

While such results may seem inevitable, even desirable as a means of sustaining cultural values, it is vital to realize that the existence of the terms contributes to the proliferation of subtle but treacherous hierarchies, accompanied as they are by various practices of distancing and degradation (Goffman, 1961). In this sense, the existence of a vocabulary of deficit is akin to the availability of weapons: their very presence creates the possibility of targets, and once pressed into action, the "less than ideal" are encouraged to enter "treatment programs," place themselves under pharmacological care, or to separate themselves from society by entering institutions. The greater the number of criteria for mental well-being, the greater number of ways in which one can be rendered inferior in comparison to others.

It is also important to note that there is nothing about one's actions that demand these terms of discrediting. The same actions can be indexed in alternative ways with far different outcomes. Through skilled language use one might reconstruct depression as "psychic incubation," anxiety as "heightened sensitivity," and Type-A freneticism as "Protestant work ethic." Such use of the language would either reverse or erase the existing hierarchies.

Community Erosion

As we find, differing terminologies invite differing courses of action. To view teenage criminality as a problem of "economic deprivation" has different policy implications than defining it as an outcome of "gang mentality" or a "deteriorated home life." Mental deficit terms, as they function in contemporary society, are shrouded in a medical mystique. They function to name diseases or afflictions. In terms of medical logic, disease or affliction requires professional diagnosis and programs of treatment. Yet, as "the afflicted" enter such programs, "the problem" is removed from its normal context of operation and reconstituted within the professional sphere. In effect, the mental health professions appropriate the process of interpersonal realignment that might otherwise occur in the non-professional context. Relations organic to the community are thereby disrupted, communication attenuated, and patterns of interdependency destroyed. In short, there is a deterioration of community life.

One may argue that processes of natural realignment are often slow, anguished, brutal or befuddled, and that life is too short to endure the "fingers that don't fit the glove." However, the result nevertheless is that problems otherwise requiring the participation of communally related persons are removed from their ecological niche. Marriage partners carry out more intimate communication with their therapists than with each other, even saving significant insights for revelation in the therapeutic hour. Parents discuss their children's problems with specialists, or send problem children to treatment centers, and thereby reduce the possibility for authentic (unselfconscious) communication with their offspring or concerned neighbors. Organizations placing alcoholic executives in treatment programs thereby reduce the kind of self-reflexive discussions that might elucidate the possible contribution of the workplace to the problem. Partners of "problem persons" are invited away into "co-dependency support groups" where they discuss the now objectified partner with strangers. In each case, tissues of communal interdependency are injured or atrophy.

This point is drawn clearly for me in recollecting my childhood experiences with Kibby, an older man who often spoke in gibberish, had no job, and often hung around with us kids to play. We were often amused by him; sometimes we avoided him, and in our childish ways we even played jokes on him. My mother and I spoke about him from time to time; she said we should be nice to him but that he was odd and that I shouldn't play with him alone. She talked as well with Kibby's mother about possible dangers and about Kibby's future. Kibby's mother talked with most of the neighbors about her son. At that time we had no vocabulary of "mental illness," no frightening stereotypes from movies and television, and no professionals to name and treat the "illness." He was just odd Kibby, and we all got along in the neighborhood. Today I suspect Kibby would be locked in an institution, "under psychiatric care," no longer a normal feature of community life.

Self-Enfeeblement

Mental deficit terms also operate so as to essentialize the nature of the person being described. They designate a characteristic of the individual that endures across time and situation, and which must be confronted if the person's actions are to be properly understood. Mental deficit terms thus inform the recipient that "the problem" is not circumscribed, limited in time and space or to a particular domain of his/her life, but is fully general. He or she carries the deficit from one situation to another, and like a birthmark or a fingerprint, as the textbooks say, the deficit will inevitably manifest itself. In effect, once people understand their actions in terms of mental deficits, they are sensitized to the problematic potential in all their activities, the ways in which they are infected or diminished. The weight of "the problem" now expands manifold; it is as inescapable as their own shadow.

At 17, Marcia Lovejoy, a woman now working to rehabilitate schizophrenics, was herself diagnosed as schizophrenic. Her doctors informed her at the time that because of her illness, she would never work, finish school, or be able to maintain satisfactory relationships with others. The situation was described as hopeless. Lovejoy compared the diagnosis with being told one has cancer. "What would it be like if nobody who got cancer got better, and they were called by their illness? If people said, 'what should we do with these cancers? Isn't it too bad. Let's send these cancers to the hospital since we can't cure them.' " (Turkington, 1985, p. 52) To be the recipient of mental deficit terminology is thus to face a potential lifetime of self-doubt.

These outcomes—social hierarchy, communal fragmentation and self-enfeeblement—do not exhaust the unfortunate outcomes of mental deficit language. Existentialist theorists have also been concerned with the way in which such language sustains a deterministic view of human action. To have a mental illness, by current standards, is to be driven by forces beyond one's control; it is to be a victim or a pawn. Thus, for the existentialist, people cease to experience their actions as voluntary (Bugental, 1965). They feel their actions to be outside the realm of choice, inevitable and unchangeable, unless they place themselves—dependently—in professional hands. Many within the mental health professions are also concerned that the language of individual deficit draws attention away from the social context essential to the creation of such problems. Mental illness language inhibits exploration of familial, occupational and socio-structural factors of possible significance. The person is blamed; the system remains unexamined. These issues too must remain in focus.

Mental Illness as a Growth Industry

Let us consider these enfeeblements in historical perspective, and particularly the correspondent growth of the mental health professions. As earlier proposed, the discourses of psychology often spring from the natural or everyday languages of the culture. In effect, they are inherited from commonplace cultural traditions. As a result, the referential or realistic quality of such language is already consensually validated. (Processes of "thought" and "emotion," for example, are worthy of professional attention because the culture already accepts them.) Yet, once absorbed by the psychological professions, such languages undergo two major transformations. First, they are *technologized*, that is, shorn of much of their connotative richness and relocated within a series of technical practices— including theoretical analysis, measurement, and experimentation. A concept such as rationality is removed from its everyday context of usage, replaced by technical terms such as "cognition" or "information processing," thrust into artificial intelligence formalizations, measured by dichotic listening devices, and submitted to experimental investigation. As the language is technologized, so it is appropriated by the profession. The language of cognition or information processing, for example, becomes the property of the profession, and the professional now lays claim to knowledge once in the common realm. The professional becomes the arbiter of what is rational or irrational, intelligent or ignorant, natural or unnatural. As people's problems become technologized, labeled and measured by the profession, the layperson is disqualified as a knower. As a consequence, one's normal sense of self as possessing knowledge, insight, and sensitivity, is undermined (Farber, 1990). In effect, those most intimately acquainted with "the problem" must give way to the dispassionate and delimited voices of an alien authority.

This appropriation of the common language, and resulting claims to superior knowledge, are furthered by a second process, one of *self-justification*. The justification for superiority in psychological matters is primarily derived from 1) the alliance of the psychological professions with the scientific tradition more generally, and 2) the broader philosophic heritage through which the sciences are made intelligible. By claiming a position within the sciences (as opposed, for example, to religion or art), the technological discourse can acquire the rhetorical weight of disciplines such as physics or chemistry. (Doesn't most of the population believe that depression exists, even when the very term is only a century old?) Any gains within any sector of the sciences stand as promissory notes for the potentials within other "scientific" domains. Further, from early Enlightenment thought to 20th century empiricist foundationalism, we have been bathed in the rhetoric that science is both rational and progressive. In effect, by claiming themselves to be a science, supported as they are by technological accoutrements, the mental health professions benefit from "reflected glory."

To illustrate the simultaneous results of both technologizing and self-justification, consider such common terms as "the blues," "sluggishness," "sadness," "punk feelings," and "unhappiness." There is a reasonably high degree of similarity among these terms, but in everyday life each has certain performative or pragmatic capacities not shared by the others. To have "the blues" has certain honorific overtones—one has "seen how it goes," "knows life as it's lived," "has been around." The phrase commands a certain degree of respect. As one commentator points out more humorously.

> You have a right to the blues if you are older than dirt, you are blind, you shot a man in Memphis, or you can't be satisfied. You have no right to the blues if you have all your teeth, you were once blind but now you can see, the man in Memphis lived, or you have a large trust fund. You can't have the blues in an office or a shopping mall, on the golf course or at a gallery opening. You can if you are trucking on the highway, in the jailhouse, an empty bed, or at the bottom of a whisky glass. Blues beverages include cheap wine, whiskey, bourbon, muddy water or nasty black coffee. The following are not blues Beverages: Perrier, Chardonnay or Snapple.

The overtones of "the blues" are not shared by terms such as "sadness," "punk" or "unhappy." To be "unhappy," for example, often suggests that there is a contrasting state that is more normal and natural, and a possible longing or hope for return. To feel "punk" suggests a transient physical condition—possibly a sleepless night or too much drink. Each terms carries with it a range of implications, and offers action possibilities not fully suggested by the alternatives. In effect, the terms are owned by the populace and serve highly variegated functions in daily life.

Yet, for the mental health professional, these terms are considered "ignorant," merely folk approximations to some essential process lying beneath. The formal term "depression" is offered as the singular replacement for the more vague and imprecise fumblings of the masses. Technical definitions of depression are developed, case studies described, scales constructed, experimental research conducted, therapeutic strategies instituted, and treatment centers established—all of which reconstitute depression as an object of professional knowledge. Because this technical work takes place within the "scientific region" of the culture, and because science is preeminently justified, the mental health professional becomes the expert about such matters. The common citizen, now informed that his or her language is "merely colloquial" and scarcely adequate, is moved to silence. The common language loses its pragmatic potential; minority group understandings of their own lives are demeaned. As such languages are usurped, they cease to serve useful functions in everyday life.

This is to say that the mental health professions operate as agencies of unbounded transformation of meaning. They feed from all the cultural sites in which talk about the mind is extant, and as the common discourses are reshaped they become the properties of the profession—creating "conversational objects" about which the professions are the experts. As Kutchins and Kirk (1997) put it, psychiatric diagnosis effectively "pathologizes everyday life." At present there is no upward limit to the process. By remaining within the scientific perspective, there is no means by which one can easily challenge the realities created from within this perspective. In effect, the system operates internally toward full absorption of the common language, and it contains no inherent means of questioning its own premises.

To place a hard edge on the discussion let us consider the growth of the mental professions over the past century within the US. This development can be considered little short of phenomenal. To illustrate, the American Psychiatric Association was founded in 1844 by 13 physicians and hospital administrators. By the end of the century the organization had grown to 377 members. At present there are over 36,000 members of the association, some 95 times the number existing at the turn of the century. As demonstrated in Fig. 4-1, the major expansion has taken place within the last 40 years. In every decade since 1940, the membership has expanded from between 138 to 188%. There is no significant indication of leveling.[24]

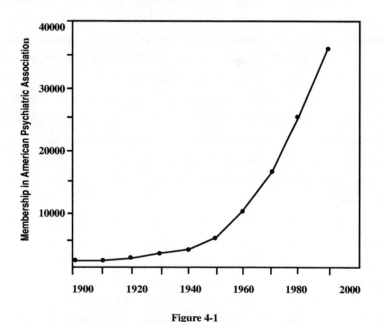

Figure 4-1
The Growth of the American Psychiatric Association

The increase in the number of practicing psychologists in the U.S. is similarly dramatic. When the American Psychological Association was founded in 1892 there were only 31 members. By 1906, the number had jumped to 181. Yet, within the 36 years that followed the membership had expanded almost 100 fold to over 3,000. In the following 22 years (between 1942 and 1966) the figure had increased again almost 20 times over, to a total of over 63,000. Of course, not all members of the Association are directly engaged in mental health pursuits, but even those who are not often lend rhetorical force to these professions. Thus, as experimentalists, intelligence testers, organizational consultants, and the like act in ways that reify mental discourse, so do they add weight to the language of the practitioner. Consider then the number of psychological personnel providing care services per 1,000,000 citizens between 1960-1983. During this period the number of psychological health providers essentially doubled within the first decade, and then trebled between 1972-1983. Again, there is no indication of a leveling of numbers, especially as therapy becomes a service provided by social work and nursing.

How are we to explain this expansion in mental health professions? Let us consider explanations favored by the two orientations toward mental discourse outlined above. For the mental realist—using the language referentially—the outlook is an optimistic one. The increment in the number of professionals represents a greater responsivity to cultural needs; existing problems are receiving greater attention. As the professions mature, it may be ventured, there is also an improvement in our capacities to distinguish among the existing array of psychological states and conditions. We know increasingly more about psychological distress, we have sharpened diagnostic distinctions, and thus can recognize problems to which we were once insensitive.

Yet, as we have also seen, the mental realist position is deeply flawed. Mental deficit terms are not tied referentially to distinctive states of the psyche. There is little to support the view that the professions have burgeoned in response to the deficient state of people's psyche, and over time have become increasingly sensitive to the failings of the mind. Let us consider, then, a pragmatic account of the trajectory. From this perspective, we find mental deficit discourse operates to generate and sustain particular ways of life. It does so first within the mental health profession. The professions themselves are highly dependent on discursive practices—the sharing of beliefs about the mind, a range of values, forms of rational justification, etc. Professional commitments depend largely on a set of shared understandings about the world and how one is to proceed. Thus, the desire of mental health professionals to increase their ranks is not a response to the world as it is, but to a shared construction of the world. At the same time, the professions could scarcely succeed in their efforts to "help society, without a public congenial to their perspectives. Sufficient segments of the culture—including prospective clients, lawmakers, the pharmacological industry, the medical profession, and insurance companies—share the language of mental illness and the belief that the professions can and should provide cures. From the pragmatic perspective there is no pattern of illness to which the professions are responding; rather, the conception of illness functions in ways that link the professional and the culture in an array of mutually supportive activities. It remains now to explore the relationship between profession and culture as it progressively expands the domain of infirmity.

The Cycle of Progressive Infirmity

As we find, the mental health professionals exist in a state of mutual symbiosis with the culture—first drawing sustenance from cultural beliefs, transforming these believes into a professional language, disseminating these views again to the culture, and relying on their incorporation into the culture for their continued sustenance. Yet, the effects of this symbiosis are increasingly alarming. In particular, there appears to be a cyclical process at work which operates to expand the domain of deficit in ever increasing degree. In effect, the very process underlying the expansion of the professions is a systematic one that feeds upon itself to engender exponentially increasing infirmity—hierarchies of discrimination, denaturalized patterns of interdependence, and an expanding arena of self-deprecation. The historical process may be viewed as one of progressive infirmity.

To explore this cycle more fully, it is useful for analytic purposes to distinguish among four separate phases. In actual practice, events in each of these phases may be confounded, with temporal ordering seldom smooth, and with exceptions at every turn. However for purposes of clarity, the cycle of progressive infirmity may be outlined as follows:

Phase 1: Deficit Translation

Let us begin at the point at which the culture accepts the possibility of "mental illness," and a profession responsible for its diagnosis and cure, a condition of ever increasing prevalence since the mid-19th century (Peeters, 1995). Under these conditions the professional confronts clients whose lives are lived out in terms of a common or everyday language. Because life management seems impossible in terms of everyday understandings the client seeks professional help—or, in effect, more "advanced," "objective," or "discerning," forms of understanding. In this context it is incumbent upon the professional to 1) furnish an alternative discourse (theoretical framework, diagnosis, etc.) for understanding the problem, and 2) translate the problem as presented in the daily language into the alternative and uncommon language of the profession. In terms of the preceding, this means that problems understood in the profane or marketplace language of the culture are translated into the sacred or professional language of mental deficit. A person whose habits of cleanliness are excessive by common standards may be labeled "obsessive compulsive," one who rests the morning in bed becomes "depressive," one who feels he is not liked is redefined as "paranoid," and so on. The client may willingly contribute to these reformulations, for not only do they assure that the professional is doing a proper job, but that the problem is well recognized and understood within the profession. However, the final outcome—translation into a professional or mental deficit vocabulary—is virtually inevitable.

Phase 2: Cultural Dissemination

Since the 18th century scientific analysis has placed great importance on classifying the various entities in its domain (e.g. animal or plant species, tables of chemical elements).[25] Emulating the natural sciences, the mental health professions have thus attempted to classify all forms of dysfunction or mental illness. As a result, not only is the "mental illness" made into a reality, but all problematic action becomes a candidate for classification as a personal illness. Further, because there are now illnesses at stake, it becomes a professional responsibility to alert the public to the fact. They must learn to recognize the signals of mental disease so that early treatment may be sought, and they should be informed of possible causes and likely cures. For example, the National Institute of Mental Health in the U.S. sends out pamphlets and provides an open website that informs the public that all the following are indicators of depression:

A sad or anxious mood
Feelings of hopelessness, pessimism
Feelings of guilt
Loss of interest or pleasure in activities
Decreased energy
Difficulty in concentrating or remembering
Inability to sleep
Oversleeping
Gaining weight

Losing weight
Restlessness
Irritability
Stomach ache, indigestion, headache

Why these are symptoms of "depression" and not something else is never made clear. Indeed, why they are symptoms at all is an open question. Is weight loss a symptom of something that is not weight loss, irritability a symptom of yet something that is not irritability? In disseminating symptom lists such as this, ordinary language is converted to a language of mental illness on a massive scale.

In the United States, the strong motive to classify and inform may be traced to the mental hygiene movement early this century. For millions of people Clifford Beers' famous volume, A Mind That Found Itself (going into 13 editions within 20 years of its publication in 1908) first served to substantiate mental illness as a phenomenon, to bring the appalling conditions of mental hospitals into the public eye, and by implication, to warn the general public of the existing threat of such illness. Coincident with its publication the National Committee for Mental Hygiene was founded, and by 1917 began publishing its national quarterly, Mental Hygiene. This magazine, along with an array of pamphlets on such topics as "childhood, the golden period for mental hygiene," "nervousness, its cause and prevention," "the movement for a mental hygiene of industry," and "the responsibility of the universities in promoting mental hygiene," attempted to bring issues of mental illness into the public eye, and to encourage major institutions (schools, industries, communities) to develop preventative programs. In the same way that signs of breast cancer, diabetes, or venereal disease should become common knowledge within the culture, it was (and is) argued, citizens should be able to recognize early symptoms of stress, alcoholism, depression and the like.

Although the mental hygiene movement is no longer visible as such, its logic has now been absorbed by the culture. Most large scale institutions do provide services for the mentally disturbed—whether in terms of health services, guidance counselors, clinical social workers, or insurance coverage for therapy. University curricula feature courses on adjustment and abnormality, national magazines and newspapers disseminate news of mental disorder (e.g. depression and its cure through chemistry) and problems of mental illness are popular fare in television dramas and soap operas. Further, the general public has sufficiently absorbed the mental hygienist mentality that books on psychological self-help are now mainstays in the publication industry. The result is a continuous insinuation of the professional language into the sphere of daily relationships.[26]

So sensitized is the culture to possible deficits that in certain quarters professionals are no longer required for the process of "enlightenment." Grass roots movements now spring up in dramatically expanding numbers, dedicated to increasing community awareness of mental deficit, to ways in which the unsuspecting contribute to such deficit, and to developing programs for the alleviation of the problems. I recently scanned the pages of a community newspaper from Santa Fe, New Mexico, to find announcements for some 14 meetings of groups dedicated to overcoming psychological deficits. One could gain help not only for obvious problems with alcohol and other drugs, but for overeating, sexual addiction, being co-dependent with sex addicts, attitudinal problems, love addiction, gay sexual compulsiveness, and proneness to debt. There were only three meetings announced for business professionals (e.g. Rotary, Kiwanis). More generally, there are now over 100 forms of twelve-step, self-help organizations, organized to treat people suffering from everything from emotionality to gambling.

Phase 3: The Cultural Construction of Illness

As vocabularies of deficit are disseminated to the culture, they become absorbed into the common language. They become part of " what everybody knows" about human behavior. In this sense, terms such as neurosis, stress, alcoholism and depression are no longer "professional property." They have been "given away" or returned by the profession to the public. Terms such as split personality, identity crisis, PMS (premenstrual syndrome), attention deficit and mid-life crisis also enjoy a high degree of popularity. And, as such terms make their way into the cultural vernacular, they become available for the construction of everyday reality. Veronica is not simply "too fat;" she has "obese eating habits;" Robert doesn't simply "hate gays," but is "homophobic;" and so on. As deficit terms become increasingly available for making the social world intelligible, that world becomes increasingly populated by deficit. Events which passed unnoticed become candidates for deficit interpretation; actions once viewed as "good and proper" can now be reconceptualized as obsessive, phobic, or repressive. Once terms such as "stress" and "occupational burnout" enter the commonsense vernacular, they become lenses through which any working professional can reexamine his/her life and find it wanting. What was valued as "active ambition" can now be reconstructed as "workaholic;" the "smart dresser" can be redefined as "narcissistic," and the "autonomous and self-directed man" becomes "defended against his emotions." As we furnish the population with hammers of mental deficit, everyone needs pounding.

Nor is it simply deficit labeling that is at stake here. For as forms of "illness" are described in the media, educational programs, public talks, and the like, the symptoms come to serve as cultural models. In effect, the culture learns *how to be* mentally ill. Consider the spread of "anorexia" and "bulimia," once "eating disorders" became publicly recognized. So fully depicted was "the illness" by the media that any discontented adolescent suddenly was furnished with a mode of expression. Similarly, depression has become such a cultural commonplace that it is virtually an invited reaction to failure, frustration or disappointment. Indeed, if one were to respond to such situations with equanimity or joy as opposed to depression, he or she might be viewed with suspicion. It is in this vein that Szasz (1960) has argued that hysteria, schizophrenia and other mental disorders represent the "impersonation" of the sick person stereotype by those confronting insoluble problems of normal living. Mental illness, in this sense, is often a form of deviant role playing, requiring a form of cultural know-how to break the rules. Sheff (1966) has made a similar case for many disorders serving as forms of social defiance. As Sheff proposes, others' reactions to the rule-breaking behavior are of enormous importance in determining whether it is finally labeled as "mental disease."

As people's actions are increasingly defined and shaped in terms of mental deficit language, there is also an increasing demand for mental health services. Counseling, weekend self-enrichment programs, and regimens of personality development represent a first line of dependence; all allow people to escape the uneasy sense that they are "not all they should be." Others may seek organized support groups for their "incest victimization," "co-dependency" or "obsession with gambling." And, of course, many enter organized programs of therapy or become institutionalized. As a result, the prevalence of "mental illness" and the associated expenditures for mental health are propelled upward. For example, in the 20 year period between 1957 and 1977 the percentage of the U.S. population using professional mental health services increased from 14% to over a quarter of the population (Kulka, Veroff and Douvan, 1979). When Chrysler Corporation insured its employees for mental health costs, the annual use of such services rose more than six times in four years ("Califano Speaks," 1984). Although mental health expenditures were minuscule during the first quarter of the century, by 1980 mental illness was the third most expensive category of health disorder in the U.S., accounting for more than $20 billion annually (Mechanic, 1987). By 1983, the costs for mental illness, exclusive of alcoholism and drug abuse, were estimated to be almost $73 billion (Harwood, Napolitano, and Kristiansen, 1983). By 1981, 23% of all hospital days in the U.S. were accounted for by mental disorders (Kiesler and Sibulkin, 1987).

Phase 4: Vocabulary Expansion

The stage is now set for the final revolution in the cycle of progressive infirmity: Further expansion in the vocabulary of deficit. As people increasingly construct their problems in the professional language, as they seek increasing help, and as the professional ranks expand in response to public demands, there are more individuals available to convert the common language into a professional language of deficit. There is no necessary requirement that such translation be conducted in terms of the existing categories of illness, and indeed there are distinct pressures on the professional for vocabulary expansion. In part, these pressures are generated from within the profession. To explore a new disorder within the mental health sciences is not unlike discovering a new star in astronomy: considerable honor may be granted to the explorer. In this sense "post-traumatic stress disorder," "identity crises," and "mid-life crisis," for example, are significant products of the "grand narrative" of scientific progress (Lyotard, 1984). They are self-proclaimed "discoveries" of the science of mental health. At the same time, new forms of disorder can be highly profitable for the practitioner, often garnering book royalties, workshop fees, corporate contracts, and/or a wealthier set of clients. In this respect such terms as "co-dependency," "stress," and "occupational burnout" have become able economic engines. The construction of Attention Deficit Disorder, and its application to populations of both children and adults, has unleashed a virtual epidemic of deficit.

On a more subtle level, there are pressures toward expansion of the professional vocabulary produced by the client population itself. As the culture absorbs the emerging argot of the profession, the role of the professional is both strengthened and threatened. If the client has already "identified the problem" in the professional language, and is sophisticated (as in many cases) about therapeutic procedures, then the status of the professional is placed in jeopardy. The sacred language has become profane. (The worst case scenario for the professional might be that people learn to diagnose and medicate themselves without professional help.) In this way there is a constant pressure placed upon the professional to "advance" understanding, to spawn "more sophisticated" terminology, and to generate new insights and forms of therapy.[27] It is not that the shift in emphasis from classic psychoanalysis to cognitive-behavior therapy is required by an increasingly sensitive understanding of mental dynamics. Indeed, each wave sets the stage for its own demise and replacement; as therapeutic vocabularies become commonly known the therapist is propelled into new modes of departure. The ever-shifting sea of therapeutic fads and fashions is no mere defect in the profession; rapid change is virtually demanded by a public whose discourse is increasingly "psychologized."

In this context it is interesting to examine the expansion of deficit terminologies. Interestingly we find here a trajectory that is suspiciously similar to those encountered in the case of mental health professionals and mental health expenditures. The concept of neurosis did not originate until the mid-18th century. In 1769 William Cullen, a Scottish physician, elucidated four major classes of morbi nervini. These included the Comota (reduced voluntary movements, with drowsiness or loss of consciousness), the Adynamiae (diminished involuntary movements), Spasmi abnormal movement of muscles), and Vesaniae (altered judgment without coma). Yet, even in 1840, with the first official attempt in the United States to tabulate mental disorders, categorization was crude. For some purposes it proved satisfactory, indeed, to use only a single category to separate the ill—including both the idiotic and insane—from the normal (Spitzer and Williams, 1985). In Germany both Kahlbaum and Kraepelin developed more extensive systems for classifying mental disease, but these were tied closely to a conception of organic origins.

With the emergence of the psychiatric profession during the early decades of the century, matters changed considerably. In particular, the attempt was made to distinguish between disturbances with a clear organic base (e.g. syphilis) and those with psychogenic origins. Thus, with the 1929 publication of Israel Wechsler's The Neuroses, a group of approximately a dozen psychological disorders were identified. With the 1938 publication of the Manual of Psychiatry and Mental Hygiene (Rosanoff, 1938), some 40 psychogenic disturbances were recognized. Many of the categories remain familiar (e.g. hysteria, dementia praecox, paranoia). More interesting from the present perspective, many of these terms have since dropped from common usage (e.g. paresthetic hysteria, autonomic hysteria); and some now seem quaint or obviously prejudicial (e.g. moral deficiency, vagabondage, misanthropy, masturbation.). In 1952, with the American Psychiatric Association's publication of the first Diagnostic and Statistical Manual of Mental Disorders it became possible to identify some 50-60 different psychogenic disturbances. By 1987—only twenty years later—the manual had gone through three revisions. With the publication of DSM IIIR the line between organic and psychogenic disturbances had also been obscured. However, using the standards of the earlier decades, in the 35 year period since the publication of the first manual, the number of recognized illnesses more than tripled (hovering between 180-200 depending on choice of definitional boundaries). At the present time, one may be classified as mentally ill by virtue of cocaine intoxication, caffeine intoxication, the use of hallucinogens, voyeurism, transvestism, sexual aversion, the inhibition of orgasm, gambling, academic problems, antisocial behavior, bereavement, and noncompliance with medical treatment. Numerous additions to the standardized nomenclature continuously appear in professional writings to the public. Consider, for example, seasonal affective disorder, stress, burnout, erotomania, the harlequin complex, and so on. Twenty years ago there was no category of illness termed Attention Deficit Hyperactivity Disorder. At present there are over 500 authoritative books and 900,000 websites that describe, explain and offer alleviation. Where are we to locate, then, the upper limits of what counts as mental disorder?

Toward Infinite Infirmity

As I am proposing, when the culture is furnished a professionally ratio-nalized language of mental deficit, and persons are increasingly under-stood in these ways, an expanded population of "patients" is created. This population, in turn, forces the profession to extend its vocabulary, and thus the array of mental deficit terms available for cultural use. More problems are thus constructed within the culture, more help sought, and the deficit discourse again inflates. One can scarcely view this cycle as smooth and undisrupted. Some schools of therapy remain committed to a single vocabulary; others have little interest in disseminating their lan-guage; some professionals attempt to speak with clients only in the com-mon language of the culture, and many popular concepts within both the culture and the profession lose currency over time (see for example, Hutschmaekers, 1989). Rather, we are speaking here of a general histori-cal drift, but one without an obvious terminus. I recently received an an-nouncement for a conference on the latest theory and research on addic-tion, announced as the "number one health and social problem facing our country today." Among the addictions to be discussed were exercise, reli-gion, eating, work, and sex. If all these activities, when pursued with intensity or gusto, are defined as diseases for which cures are required, there seems little that can withstand enfeebling translation.

It is also important to realize that in the past decade the upward spi-raling of mental illness and its enfeebling effects has been dramatically intensified. This intensification is due to the addition of three new parties to the process, the psychopharmacology industry, managed care programs and neurological research. In the first instance, the pharmacology indus-try has been enormously successful in marketing drugs that promise to alleviate most forms of daily suffering (anxiety, social phobias, unhappi-ness, tension, distress). I will take up the dramatic expansion in pharma-cological "cures" and the relationship to neurological research in the next chapter. For now it is important to note that the use of drugs to treat un-happiness has been additionally favored by the managed care movement in hospital administration. In an effort to reduce expenditures managed care has favored drugs over "talking cures" simply because it is more economical to dispense pills than pay for therapist time. By encouraging drug centered treatment, managed care programs also send a message to therapeutic practitioners more generally: if you wish to sustain a practice supported by insurance programs, it is essentially to shift to drug cen-tered treatments.[28] The result has been that organizations such as the American Psychological Association, have mounted intense programs to license their therapists to prescribe "meds" for their "patients." Such pro-grams are now achieving success, and within the next decade we can anticipate a dramatic increase in both the number of prescribing practi-tioners, and naturally, the percentage of the population dependent on drugs to "get them through the day."

There is an important sense in which the average citizen today faces a trap door into a land from which exit is difficult. There are at least three institutions of substantial size and means coordinating their efforts to ef-fectively "seduce" people into mental illness. As day to day problems of living are progressively translated into the authoritative discourse of mental illness, and drugs are offered as a secure means to restoring happiness, the attraction of drug centered "cures" is obvious. In a broad sense one might say that pharmacology is now taking the place of religion as the favored means of achieving salvation on earth.[29] Psychotherapy is rapidly becoming a bedside manner for drug dispensing.

In spite of my accusatory tone I am not ultimately attempting to allo-cate blame. For the most part this infirming of the culture is a byproduct of earnest and humane attempts to enhance the quality of people's lives and to render the process of treatment more organized and economical. And too, there are people whose suffering has been enormously allevi-ated by 1) the sense that they have a recognizable illness about which there is expert knowledge, and 2) pharmaceutical passification.[30] Everyone is attempting to "do good" within their professional niche for people who suffer and seek help. But in my view, while a minority is well served, the "sum of the parts" is catastrophic for the society more generally. The pattern is not dissimilar to that found in both the medical and legal professions—with earnest and well intended actions leading to increased medical needs and expenditures in the first instance and burgeoning litigation in the other. However, to the extent that the mental health professions, managed care providers and the pharmacological industry are concerned with the quality of cultural life, discussion of progressive infirmity should become focal. Are there important limitations to the above arguments; are there signs of a leveling effect; are there means of reducing the proliferation of enfeebling discourse? All are questions of broad significance, and all deserve concerted attention.

Steps Toward an Exit

Finally I wish to consider the question of how we might terminate the cycle of infirmity. There are critics of the mental health profession who simply wish to see the establishment abandoned. I see this alternative as neither realistic nor desirable. In many respects, the professions are essential in providing the kinds of human supports that are diminishing within the family and community spheres. Others wish to see the basic biases corrected—to remove prejudices, misclaims, and resulting inhumanities. However, the impulse to correct existing practices remains largely lodged in the realist view of mental events, and the belief that there can be objectively correct accounts of the interior world. The arguments against this view have already been treated.

I have no quick and simple solution for terminating the cycle of deficit outlined here. However, I do feel two important moves are essential:

- *Remove the requirement for deficit diagnosis.* In my view the first and most obvious means of attenuating the spiral of deficit is to break the link between deficit language and medical insurance payments. There is no evidence that treatment success depends on psychodiagnostic categorization. Yet, so long as insurance coverage is dependent on therapists placing their clients into illness categories, deficit labeling will continue to expand. There are alternatives to psychiatric diagnosis. In many countries insurance payments do not require DSM designations. In Finland and Norway enormous success has been achieved through the use of multi-party dialogue (Seikulla et al., 1995) as opposed to singular designations of disease. Rather than relying on the single view of a psychiatrist, meetings are arranged in which possibly the parents, a social worker, a teacher, a clergy member and the "designated patient" participate with the psychiatrist in understanding the nature of the problem and possible forms of alleviation. The result has been a dramatic decrease in diagnosed mental illness and the number of hospital beds occupied.
- As I will argue in the next chapter, significant change may ultimately depend on litigation against sectors of the mental health professions. To label human problems as "mental illness" can not only have injurious consequences for the suffering, but for the culture as a whole. It is not only that such constructions are groundless, but they are specious parallels to our understanding of biological illness. Unlike biological illnesses such as malaria, diabetes, or small pox there are few instances in which one can identify 1) the starting period of the disease, 2) the means by which it is transmitted or otherwise originates, or 3) its termination. If there are legal restrictions placed on dispensing pharmaceuticals and claims for medical cures, there should be no less protection against claims and cures of mental health professionals. If litigation is to

proceed, invaluable will be the vast numbers who see themselves as victimized or abused by the system. The anti-psychiatry movement may be the best resource for change.[31]

- *Develop and support alternative constructions.* Therapists themselves may also work with their clients to develop more positive or promising constructions of their condition. There is momentum here, not only evidenced in preceding chapters, but as well by constructivist and constructionist therapists more generally (see Neimeyer and Raskin, 2000). Such efforts should also be combined with expanding multi-cultural discussion of mental illness classification. There are enormous differences among sub-cultures in the meaning attached to "problems," (see Kutchins and Kirck, 1997), and in this respect such offerings may form contributions to reconstruction. Finally, therapists should lend their efforts to various ex-patient groups attempting to reconceptualize their "illnesses." There are groups of "ex-schizophrenics," for example, who are able to re-draw the nature of their problem. As they see it, they do not have an illness, but special sensitivities. They are more highly sensitive to the various tensions inherent in human relations than others, and thus less able to cope. Their problem is not being sick, but having too much of a good thing. Similarly there are support groups that celebrate the hearing of multiple voices, and the possession of multiple personalities. Why should these be illnesses; one might indeed see them as assets. Support and advocacy of such groups is essential.[32]

These are scarcely the only alternatives to bringing the spiral of deficit under control. And, whatever forward looking moves are made in policy and practice must be coupled with a concern for the enormous impact of the bio/pharma movement on both our understanding and treatment of human problems. It is to these latter issues we turn in the next chapter.

5

The Neurobiological Turn: Salvation Or Devastation?

Most Americans, and even many doctors, have never heard of social anxiety disorder, and it affects more than 5 million Americans, according to the National Institute of Mental Health. Drug companies, eager to expand their markets, are now spotlighting the disorder—and advertising medications to treat it....Technology is now helping to pinpoint changes in socially anxious brains.

<u>Newsweek</u>, July 2003

If there is one hallmark of the mental health professions since their very beginnings, it has been conflict. Not only was conflict a dominant motif within Freud's privileged circle of colleagues, but since that time the professions have come to resemble a virtual battlefield of competing schools, practices, ideals, and truths. Yet, there is now a gathering of forces into two major camps, and far more hangs in the balance than the survival one orientation as opposed to another. At the broadest level I am speaking here of a competition between two major ways of understanding human functioning, their resulting forms of practice and policy, and their impact on the culture more broadly. On the one side are professionals who emphasize the natural or biological roots of human behavior, and on the other those who are concerned with the cultural constitution of human action. From the former standpoint, rigorous diagnostics, neurological research, managed care, and pharmacology are favored routes to "curing mental illness." From the latter standpoint, not only are there enormous dangers inherent in this naturalist orientation, but there is rampant blindness to the cultural process in which human suffering is embedded, and the kinds of therapeutic processes essential to bringing about change. How are we to respond to this conflict? Much hangs in the balance.

Given the constructionist orientation developed in the preceding chapters, you might readily surmise my strong preference for a more culturally sensitive orientation to human suffering. However, because of the enormous outpouring of neuroscience research on psychological processes, the associated burgeoning in psychopharmacological prescriptions, and the broad embracing of these movements by the managed care system, a more responsible assay is invited. It is not enough to view with alarm the sweeping changes occurring in the mental health establishment. More measured and incisive arguments are required.

In what follows I first wish to consider some of the major repercussions of the neurobiological movement in today's world of therapeutic practice. I then turn to neurological inquiry into psychological processes. To what extent does such research warrant or support a shift toward a biological orientation in mental health practices? Is there sufficient support for the neurological orientation to offset the various costs? Finding such support quite negligible, I will explore several important implications for policy and practice.

The reader should be sensitized in advance to two aspects of this analysis. First, while there are many who not unwisely conclude that both biological and cultural factors play a part in "mental illness," in what follows I will place the two positions in an antagonistic relationship. It is important at this juncture to gain clarity on what is taking place in the neuro/biological move. Simply fusing the positions leaves many issues unaddressed. Second, in this analysis I do not ultimately mean to objectify either the neuro/biological or cultural orientations. That is, both orientations construct the world in their own particular ways. However, much hangs on these constructions in terms of their impact on cultural life. It is the consequences that concern me most.

The Emerging Tragedy

While resistance to the bio-medical model of mental suffering has long been robust, recent advances in research have dramatically shifted the momentum. Relying on various developments in brain scanning technology, research consistently reveals what appear to be the neural bases of wide ranging behavior. To the extent that such research can pinpoint the neural basis of what are commonly viewed as psychological disorders, strong support is provided for 1) the diagnostic categorization of mental illness, 2) the development of pharmacological treatments for such illnesses, and 3) the efficient dispensing of treatment to the afflicted. If "mental problems" are essentially biological problems in disguise, then the same diagnostic precision pursued by the medical profession should be installed in therapeutic professions. If abnormal behavior can be traced to particular brain states, then treatment of abnormality must primarily focus on alteration of neural conditions. Such alterations can be achieved least intrusively and most dependably through biochemistry. And, if problems in human behavior are essentially biological, then any form of treatment that is non-biological fails to be cost effective. To effectively manage care, pharmacological treatment should ultimately replace the more expensive and less relevant forms of "talk therapy."

In the preceding chapter I took up the societally injurious consequences of the trend toward unwarranted and unbridled psychodiagnosis. Here I shall confine myself to the societal repercussions of the neurobiological program more specifically, and its alliance with pharmacological treatment and managed care programs.

Toward a Drug Dependent Culture

Perhaps the most dramatic cultural transformation favored by the biologizing of human suffering is the shift from culturally sensitive "talking cures," to psychopharmacology. Thirty years ago there were relatively few anti-psychotic drugs available, and drug treatments were typically limited to the severely impaired. In 1970 there were approximately 150,000 mental health cases treated pharmacologically in the U.S. By the year 2,000 the number jumped to between 9-10 million. More than half the cases treated by psychotropic drugs were school children. At the publication of the present volume, Amazon lists almost 6,000 books on the subject of psychopharmacology. The browser of this list will also have a difficult time locating books that are critical—or even cautious—about the use of drugs in psychiatric practice.

The impact of this movement on the individual were recently made clear to me by by a Florida therapist, Phillip Sinaikin (2004):

> *A 60 year old divorced female was referred to me by a fellow psychiatrist who was leaving private practice. The frazzled looking woman informed me that she is diagnosed as a rapid-cycling biopolar and then presented me with a list of her current medications. She was being treated with Lamictal (an anticonvulsant) 100 mg three times a day, Alpazolam (a tranquilizer) 1 mg three times a day, Celexa (an antdepressant) 40 mg per day, Wellbutrin (an antidpressent) 150 mg twice a day, Seroquel (an antipsychotic) 300 mg at bedtime, Fiorinol (a barbiturate containing pain pill) up to 4 a day and finally Ritalin (an amphetamine stimulant) 20 mg three times a day. That is 17 pills a day!...Asked about her current supply of medications, she didn't know what she had or needed. All she knew for certain was that she was out of Ritalin and needed a refill. By that time, the hour allotted for her intake was up. So, do I give her a refill and further legitimize what I view as an irrational and dangerous diagnostic conceptualization and treatment plan by her previous psychiatrist? And if I choose not to, what do I do?* (p. 38)

There is more to the pharmacological turn than its impact on the suffering client. There are also economic and cultural implications of enormous proportion. In economic terms, consider the growth of the major antidepressant, Prozac. According to a <u>Newsweek</u> (March 26, 1990) report, a year after the drug was introduced to the market sales reached $125 million. One year later (1989) the sales had almost tripled to $350 million. By 2002, Prozac was a $12 billion industry! At present there are over 25 million prescriptions for Prozac (or its generic equivalent) in the US alone. A similar number of prescriptions are written for Zoloft, a close cousin, and another 25 million for a combination of other competitors. (New York Times, June 30, 2002). Consider that at the turn of the century, depression was virtually non-existent as a cultural concern. Currently there are now over 33 million websites devoted to depression.

One may read such figures in three equally unsettling ways. In the first case, they represent increased expenditures on mental health. Given the unwarranted practices of diagnosis, we must confront the possibility that as a culture we are needlessly constructing the population in ways that increasingly expand public expenditures. In this sense, drug cures are not enabling managed care programs to reduce health care costs as anticipated, but are working cooperatively to produce exponentially increasing expenditures. One may also read these economic figures in terms of profits to the pharmaceutical industry. Given the unfettered expansion of psychodiagnostic categories and the willingness of the society to "trust the experts," future profits are almost guaranteed. The availability of profit also means the launching of additional research and the availability of still further drugs, and the marketing of these drugs to both mental health professionals and the public. Again we confront an unending spiral. Finally, one may see these figures in terms of the capacity of the pharmaceutical industry to discourage or block any legislation that would threaten profitability. With the enormous funds available to the industry, the power of the lobbies also increases. Help from the government becomes ever less likely.

One must ultimately inquire into the message which the routinizing of drug treatment sends to the culture at large. Essentially the culture is informed by professional authorities that drugs are the answer to common problems of human living. If one is deeply grieving, anxious about work, distressed by failure, frightened of social life, unable to stop working, worried about homoerotic tendencies, or is growing too thin, drugs are the answer. In previous times we human beings have acquired individual coping strategies or relied upon one another. These cultural resources for resiliency are increasingly under threat. In effect, the neurobiological shift increases dependence of the culture on artificial supports for normal life. Psychopharmacology takes its place along side drugs for sleeping, sexual arousal, increasing athletic prowess, and euphoric pleasure. A recent cartoon depicted a little leaguer asking a druggist if he had something that could help him hit home runs. We are approaching a condition in which we will turn to the medicine cabinet in order to "get through" a normal day.

Cultural Myopia

To the extent that we attribute the problems of the individual to neurobiological conditions, concern for the cultural context fades from view. In certain degree, the medical model of illness, of which the neurobiological orientation to human suffering is a descendent, shares in this problem. The medical profession is deeply engaged in searching for a cure for various diseases, but it is the task of other professions (such as public health and epidemiology) to consider means of changing sexual practices to reduce the spread of the virus. But in the case of what passes for mental illness, the case for neglecting application is far more serious. There are two major issues to consider:

Of primary importance, there is substantial reason to believe that much of what passes as mental illness is sociogenic in origin. This is so in two important ways. First, the origins of most human suffering are lodged within traditions of cultural meaning. Experiences of personal failure, loss of control, deficient self confidence, shame, humiliation, loss of love, the death of an intimate, and fear of evaluation, for example, are all common topics addressed to therapists by suffering patients. Yet, all of these topics exist only within particular traditions of meaning. For example, there is nothing about personal failure that is itself demanding of anguish.

In fact, we experience myriad failures toward which we are relatively indifferent (e.g. losing at various games), and the importance we attach to others (e.g. failing at marriage) is owing entirely to the value placed on such events by the surrounding culture. Similarly, it is only in a culture that places a value on autonomy or the personal control of outcomes that losing control is a reason for depression. Even in many Western sub-cultures there is a strong value conferred on placing one's destiny in the hands of a deity. To the extent that personal problems are embedded within processes of cultural meaning, the primary emphasis should be placed on movement within these processes. Neurobiology is largely irrelevant.

This emphasis on culture is also important because it opens up consideration of the social conditions in which we live our lives. As Karen Horney (1950) once proposed, many of our institutions are themselves sources of anxiety. Conditions of intense competition, high professional insecurity, information overload, poverty, and oppression will all be reflected in degrees of human suffering. To treat such suffering as biological in nature is not only to blind oneself to the proper origins, but to insure that the therapeutic profession is left only to treat the effects of our problems and never the cause.

Such arguments have long been fortified by cross-cultural, historical and demographic studies of mental illness. In the cultural case we find broad and significant differences in what is counted as deviant in cultural life, how it is understood, and the cultural practices in which it is embedded (see for example, Al-Issa, 1995). The fact that some forms of activity viewed as "mental illness" in the American cultural setting scarcely occur in others, is a strong argument against a biological disease model. Coupled with significant cultural differences are significant accounts of historical changes in what is constructed or defined as mental illness (see, for example, Hacking, 1985; Lerman, 1996; Hepworth, 1999). And in terms of demographics, the fact that depression is most disproportionately located in lower class populations, in women, and in the aged is difficult to justify in terms of a disease model of depression. For example, people in the lowest economic strata in the US are three times more likely to be diagnosed with a mental disorder. Strong arguments for the contagiousness of mental disease have never been put forward, and why such groups should be more genetically prone to mental illness remains a mystery. However, the fact that all such groups live under circumstances of high stress, provides a ready explanation in terms of cultural genesis.

There is a second way in which the attribution of anguish to neuro/biological causes suppresses concern with the socio-cultural issues. In this case attention turns to the very definition of "mental illness." As I proposed in the preceding chapter, there has been an exponential expansion in the labeling of undesirable behavior as "mental illness." If our definitional systems were otherwise, such behavior would not count as illness, and new questions could be asked about the source of its undesirability. For example, there is nothing inherently "ill" about a highly active child, and the primary reason for the label resides in inability of teachers to effectively carry out their task. In effect, the teacher's suffering is re-directed to the child, and labeled as an illness for which pharmacology is the answer. Virtually no attention is thus directed to practices of teaching more optimally suited for highly varied student proclivities, or the cultural conditions that favor hyper-activity (e.g. electronic games).

Emily Martin (2000) argues that indeed some forms of activity at one time defined as mentally ill are now becoming valued:

Mania is becoming highly valued in the workplace. If concepts of the ideal person are changing in such contexts as work, life and value, demanding restless change and development of the person at all times, in all realms, then manic depression might readily come to be regarded as   normal—even ideal—for the human condition under these historically specific circumstances. (p. 190)

Closely related to the cultural construction of illness is the impact of disease diagnosis on those who are treated. The individual labeled as mentally ill, takes on a dimension of self-doubt for which there is no ultimate termination. Unlike physical illnesses, in which one can typically identify the onset and termination, the label of mental illness essentially remains forever. Because there are no unambiguous indicators of beginning or end, there is no way one can be certain that the "illness" is not influencing his or her actions in some devious way, or is there hovering in the wings. A strong case can be made for much that counts as mental illness being *iatrogenic* in character, that is a form of suffering created through the very practices of diagnosis and treatment. At least 41,000 websites now attest to this possibility. Inquiry into all these matters is pushed aside in the turn to the neurobiological model.[1]

Mechanical Care

To the extent that problems of human suffering can be attributed to biological causes, then the medical model of treatment is invited. Among the traditional criteria for medical treatment are rapidity, efficacy, and efficiency. The most effective treatment of the body should be provided as rapidly as possible for the least cost. Although we are beginning to understand the limits of medical care bereft of concern for the human conditions of illness (Bolen, 1996; Murphy, 1997), the medical model is deeply problematic when applied to problems of unspecified biological origin. In the case of physical illness, the patient's anguish typically originates in the illness itself (e.g. pain, incapacity in physical functioning); personal problems are secondary. When people ask for psychotherapeutic help, their problems are almost invariably personal, and physical pain infrequent. To treat the personal problems as secondary, if not irrelevant, is a virtual negation of *human* being as such. Critical issues of human social existence are trivialized in favor of drug treatments that effectively render the individual insensitive to such issues. Donald (2001) describes the "Wal-Marting of American psychiatry," "the movement toward mindless cost control measures, and the associated vision of human beings as generic and interchangeable." In the same vein, Cushman and Gilford

(2000) see the managed care of mental suffering as negating the significance of human experience, and replacing a concern with individual
meaning with impersonal quantification. As they see it, the move toward
managed care brings with it a fundamental change in our definition of
what it is to be human. The humanistic vision gives way to a materialist
instrumentalism.

The Erosion of Multi-Party Dialogue

In his pivotal volume, Legitimation Crisis, the German philosopher,
Jurgen Habermas brought critical attention to the limitations of instrumental reasoning. Such reasoning is centrally concerned with how various ends can most practically be achieved. How can we build a faster
computer, improve law enforcement, or combat terrorism more effectively? And yet, argues Habermas, the headlong thrust toward imple-
menting ends typically subverts debate over the values underlying such
efforts. In fighting terrorism, for example, we neglect inquiry into underlying issues of cultural differences, value relativism, and our own
contribution to the phenomenon.

The mental health professions have a long tradition of instrumental
reasoning. The neurobiological turn serves only to intensify such an orientation. The purported identification of brain state indicators of mental
illness, and the accompanying expansion of pharmaceutical cures, constitutes a strong invitation for more experimentation, more facts, and
greater efficacy. Yet, as we launch inquiry into effective practices, removed from consciousness are significant differences in views and values about such issues as defining illness, who gains and loses from such
definitions, and the broad societal implications of drug prescriptions. In
the quest for the goal, we no longer ask about the value of the goal and its
potential for injury.

Thus, to launch broad-scale inquiry into the neurological basis of
mental illness or optimal drug dosages for cure is not simply the quest for

scientifically neutral knowledge. Rather, the very presumption that non-normal behavior or various forms of human suffering constitute "illnesses" is already value saturated. As Sadler's (2002) important effort makes quite clear, the DSM illness categories are themselves implicit statements of what constitutes the "good society." When Peter Kramer (2005) rails against those who would romanticize depression by seeing it as a route to creativity and deeper understanding, he is essentially making a moral claim: those who find value in "feeling down" do not contribute to the good society as he defines it. This is not to argue against the values inherent in either the DSM or to privilege happiness over the blues. However, what is essential is to bring these biases to light, and to project them into the broader cultural dialogues on the nature of the good society. The failure to acknowledge and debate is little short of an oppressive silencing of the diverse sub-cultures making up the society.

The Limits of Neuroscience

The perils outlined here are unsettling primarily to the extent that the neuro/biological orientation is inadequate in either explaining or treating what we commonly term "mental illness." If indeed there were outstanding evidence in support of the orientation, we might simply have to reconcile ourselves with a certain degree of collateral damage. We might have to content ourselves with dramatic increases in drug use, less humane health care, inattention to cultural context of human suffering, and questions of the good. So, we may well wish to ask, what is the evidence?

While a full review of all the biological evidence is beyond the scope of this chapter, I do wish to take up the recent spate of neurologically centered research. It is this research that has come to provide the most dramatic support to the biological orientation. As indicated earlier, such research has been particularly spurred by the development of various technologies (e.g. MRI, PET, EEG, MEG) for scanning brain activity. Thus, as subjects are engaged in various activities—problem solving, remembering, bargaining, watching films, meditating, and so on, measures can be taken of heightened neuro/chemical activity in various areas of the brain. The typical attempt is to locate those areas of the brain that are specific to a given psychological state or behavior.

Such research is dramatic in implication because it seems to reveal the neural basis of the state or activity in question. In the field of mental health, the drama is particularly powerful. Rather than relying on the highly ambiguous diagnostic criteria outlined in the DSM, brain scans reveal the different locations in the brain implicated in various pathological states. Differences in brain functioning, let's say, between normal samples in comparison to those diagnosed as schizophrenic or bi-polar, directly demonstrate the locus of pathology. The guess-work is finished.

Given this general logic, and the resulting cornucopia of research findings, what reasons are there for pause? On what grounds, if any, should we resist what appear to be reasonable and empirically grounded proposals? In my remarks I will put aside the notorious methodological problems that inhabit such research. There are enormous problems, for example, in isolating from the continuous flow of neurological change a singular state to which a given behavior can legitimately be attributed. And, given the differing ways in which human brains can react to the same external conditions, locating an identical state across populations of any kind is hazardous. One can only imagine the theory invested sorting and sifting of visual data that must occur. Rather, my concern here is with major flaws in the logic underlying the attempt to locate neural bases of human problems:

Plasticity and the Return of Culture

To say that a given brain state is the underlying basis of a given problem is to specify the brain as the causal source. Thus, if the source of the problem is fixed within the nervous system, then therapeutic intervention must focus on alteration of the nervous system. By analogy, if one's automobile fails to function properly, engine repair may be required. However, this argument is reasonable only to the extent that it is the structure of the machinery in itself that is at fault. If the failure of the machinery can be traced to a prior cause—falling outside its confines—then correcting the machinery is only a temporary and possibly futile effort. If one's engine does not function properly because one has failed to replenish its oil, then attention must be directed to the oil supply and not the properties of the engine.

This latter possibility is most obviously relevant in those brain studies attempting to isolate a singular process from an ongoing stream. Here, for example, researchers focus on the neural processes "responsible for" memory, problem solving, trust, meditation, prayer, political preferences, and the like. In all such cases, however, various experimental manipulations or instructions are required to bring the state of the brain into its condition. To create a brain state indicative of "distrust," for example, requires that circumstances of distrust are established in the laboratory. Thus, the circumstances, it may be said, bring the state into existence. It is not the brain condition that is the basis of distrust, but the conditions of distrust that bring about the brain state.

A more compelling case for neural origins is found in research comparing brain scans of people who are chronically ill with those who are deemed normal. Here researchers compare, for example, schizophrenic, bi-polar, ADHD, or obsessive compulsive samples with "normals." Yet, while such research often reveals differences, the question of cause still remains. To what extent is it the brain condition that gives rise to the symptoms, as opposed to a preceding condition that brings about the brain condition? If one lives for many years under oppressive, stressful, hopeless, or anxiety provoking conditions, it is possible that cortical connections are altered. However, we may ask, could we not be more effective by attending to the precipitating conditions as opposed to their results?

It is at this point that an enormous body of evidence for neural plasticity becomes relevant. As wide-ranging research has demonstrated, the brain continues to reorganize itself by forming new neural connections throughout life. For one, neurons can be developed to compensate for injury. Existing neural pathways that are inactive or used for other purposes show the ability to take over and carry out functions lost to degeneration. Further, neurogenesis (the development of new nerve cells) enables the individual to adjust to new situations or changes in the environment. Although accelerated in the pre-natal period, neurogenesis continues into old age. To the extent that plasticity prevails, we may abandon the view that the brain serves as the chief determinant of cultural action; rather, it is the cultural context that determines how the brain will function.

To the extent that the plasticity explanation is reasonable, then the reliance on pharmacological "cures to mental illness" is also thrown into significant question. If states of what we call "depression" (along with associated neural markers) are not inherent in biology, but are created culturally, then pharmacological cure is akin to tinkering with the engine to cure the problems of oil depletion. To be sure, medications may enable one to cope with oppressive or stressful conditions. If properly sedated, the conditions are less arousing. However, without intervention into the conditions, or enhancement of the person's resiliency skills, we succeed only in contributing to a culture of zombies.

Interpretation Bias: The Cultural Reading of the Brain

Brain scan studies have been welcomed with enthusiasm by many mental health professionals because they seem to provide an answer to the plaguing problem of inference. This is the problem of inferring the existence of a psychological condition (e.g. depression) from over behavior (e.g. inability to sleep). We guess about the nature of "mental" illness by its symptoms, and we attempt to validate our inferences through multiple expressions. For example, while inability to sleep may not guarantee that a person is depressed, that the person says he thinks of suicide strengthens the inference. However, such seeming validations are ultimately problematic, as they too remain inferential. Thus, an individual may feel suicidal precisely because he is so exhausted from lack of sleep that he cannot cope. Depression may be irrelevant. Any interpretation remains suspended, then, on a network of ultimately unwarranted and hypothetical interpretations.

Do brain scan data solve this notorious problem of inference? Let us take a closer look. Consider again the dilemma of psychological diagnosis: we are presented with a collection of expressions that we classify as symptoms of an underlying condition, but we have no access to the causal condition itself. In effect, we have been forced to speculate that loss of appetite, lack of sleep, and feelings of hopelessness are symptoms of an underlying state of depression. We now observe the neural condition of the person we have shakily diagnosed as depressed. We succeed in locating a neural condition unique to this population. Yet, we may ask, how can we determine that the observed state of the brain is in fact "depression?" Why, is it not simply a neural correlate of sleeplessness, appetite loss, or feelings of helplessness?" Or for that matter, how could we determine that the neural state is not one of "spiritual malaise," "anger," "withdrawal from oppressive conditions," or "cognitive integration and regrouping?"

In effect, brain scan data do not solve the problem of inference, but simply remove it from one site of ignorance to another. Brain scans do not speak for themselves. To read them as evidence of depression, deceit, trust, empathy, political preferences, and so on is little more than exercising a sub-cultural bias. And, as argued in the preceding chapter, it is precisely the reading of the mind in terms of "mental illness" that contributes to the massive diseasing of the population.

Winks and Blinks: The Impossibility of Reductionism

Neurological description is optimally employed in giving accounts of specific observations of the brain. Brain state terms may legitimately be employed to explain various behavioral movements of the body, when neurological conditions are constituents of the movements themselves. Thus, to the extent that there are lesions in the motor cortex I may not be able to move my arms or fingers. The condition of the brain is neurologically linked to the bodily movement. It is thus that the study of the neural mechanisms involved in aphasia, downs syndrome, or brain tumors may serve vitally useful purposes. We are speaking in each case of a contiguous neurological system.

Yet, we encounter severe problems when we attempt to apply the neural model to what we might call "meaningful actions" within the culture. In carrying out cultural life, it is useful to describe various people as "aggressive," "moral," "helpful," "dishonest," "humorous" and the like. We may usefully describe our emotional expressions as "anger," "happiness," "love," or "anxiety." Yet, while such discourse is critical to living an effective life within the culture, none of these descriptors is linked to determinate movements of the body. To illustrate, consider the following bodily movement: my hand takes the shape of a fist, and I move my index finger back and forth. To be sure, there is a neurological basis for the spatio-temporal movements of the finger. But, our cultural descriptors are linked only partially and contestably to movements of the body. If the movement of the finger is pulling the trigger or a gun aimed at another person, our description is far different than if the finger is used to beckon us to the bedroom. And it is crucial for effective cultural life to make a distinction between "murder" and "seduction." The scope of neurological expertise ends with the account of the bodily movement; it is mute with respect to cultural meaning. Neurology can tell us much about the blink of the eye, but nothing about the wink.

On this account, neurological accounts are highly limited with respect to most activity that we describe as mentally ill. Consider an eight year old boy walking about the classroom while the teacher is talking. We may account for the specific movements of the body neurologically. But these movements are not themselves significant. The boy could have walked slowly or rapidly, haltingly or smoothly, stamping his feet or not. The precise movements are not at all important. What is important in labeling the behavior a symptom of attention deficit is that they are inappropriate in the classroom setting. In the same way, activities described as compulsive, phobic, or masochistic have no determinate neural correlates. More broadly we may say that most of the behavioral descriptions employed in the DSM cannot be described in neural terms. The behaviors in question may be infinite in their variation; it is the cultural meaning that enables us to identify them and it is working within these systems of meaning that change may effectively be accomplished.

Proposals for a More Promising Future

To be sure, my arguments here are dedicated to illuminating the shortcomings of the neurobiological movement in mental health. In my view, the claims made for the movement—both professionally and in the public media—are virtually without critical self-reflection. Perhaps the present account can contribute to a much needed dialogue. In spite of my critique, I am not at all proposing a termination of neurobiological inquiry into problems of human suffering or the pharmacological treatments with which such inquiry is identified. However, if the current trajectory in our understanding of human problems and their treatment is continued, we are collectively bringing about a cultural disaster. In my view it is first essential to slow the pace of the neurobiological juggernaut, and as we do so to nurture the kinds of careful assessments that can yield more reasonable and culturally protective policies and practices. Three initiatives seem especially demanding of attention:

Restrict the Pharmacological Alternative

At the present time we are witnessing an exponential increment in drug prescriptions for therapeutic clients. Under the continuing influence of the pharmacological industry and managed care programs to expand profit margins, there is little reason to suspect a diminishing. Indeed, given the increasingly successful attempts of other professions, such as clinical psychology, to gain prescription privileges, we might anticipate an expansion in drug usage. And, given the continuous conversion of common problems in living to diagnostic categories (described in the previous chapter), there is no upward limit in sight.

It seems to me that of immediate importance are initiatives that would place significant restrictions on drug prescriptions. Policies might be developed that would place medications as a secondary form of treatment, essential only in serious conditions. I would like to think that the psychiatric profession harbors a sufficient sense of dedication to the public good that movements toward responsible treatment would originate there. At the same time, such a movement is not likely to be successful without involving both the institutions of managed care and the insurance companies. There are not only complex financial problems to address, but issues of malpractice litigation attendant upon *failure* to administer drugs.

Awaiting major shifts in policy, two additional ends are more easily in reach. First, policies of full disclosure are essential before clients are placed on medication. The side-effects of many existing meds are notorious (see, for example, Breggin, 1994, 2000; Breggin and Breggin, 1995). It is not only the range and seriousness of these side-effects that should be clarified, but the possible trajectories of drug use that are possible. The likely failure, re-adjustments, and compounding of drugs over time should be clarified. That one may soon find themselves taking 17 pills a day is a fact that might well deter many from embarking on the pharmaceutical journey. Highly recommended in this case would be the development of web-sites that spell out for therapy clients the impact of medications on their lives.[1] The increment in superficial mood or coping capacity is always purchased at a cost to well-being. These costs should become matters of public knowledge.

Coupled with responsible warning practices, programs of drug reduction are vitally needed. While drug prescriptions can be obtained with the virtual ease of over-the-counter purchasing, means of exiting regimens of drug usage are little developed. On the contrary, in many quarters of psychiatry the presumption prevails that psychiatric illness is a life-time affair. When we consider the inability to locate a medical infirmity, such a presumption invites accusations of gross irresponsibility. Again, we find a condemning contrast with traditional medical practice. To cure a medical condition and leave the patient with a life-long prescription to the curative would be unconscionable. Most importantly, however, inventive programs are needed for reducing and ultimately eliminating drug dependency. At present, most "patients" must find their own way of eliminating drug dependency. Many are heroic in this respect; others suffer greatly (Lehmann, 2004). The professional challenge—both practical and moral—is clear.

Prioritize Cultural Meaning

To be sure, it is essential to explore more thoroughly the nexus of cultural and biological forces giving rise to the suffering confronted by mental health professionals. I have little doubt that there are numerous cases of suffering for which a clearly identifiable physical cause may be located and for which a medical cure is appropriate. However, the mere location of neurological correlates to suffering provides no basis at all for presuming a medical illness. Nor does the fact that pharmaceuticals can successfully reduce such suffering add supporting evidence to the medical approach. Rather, to the extent that they are successful, drugs appear primarily to sedate and suppress. The ultimate cause of the suffering remains unexplored. In the medical case, one would scarcely consider reducing conscious suffering at the expense of determining the cause. Indeed, such a practice would typically prove fatal for the patient as the disease would intensify. (The fact that there is no record of fatalities resulting from symptom treatment in the world of mental health again suggests that we are not dealing with a biological illness.)

In my view, strong investments should be made into forms of therapy and related practices that are 1) maximally sensitive to cultural meaning systems and/or 2) engender skills in navigating a world of conflict, oppression, and threat. Required in therapy is an abiding concern with the thoughts, feelings, memories, fantasies, and so on through which the world and self are understood (Cushman, 1995). While classic psychoanalysis held that this realm of personal meaning was largely hidden by repression, object relations theory and feminist psychoanalytic theory have now brought it into more ready accessibility (see, for example, Spence, 1982; Mitchell, 1993) In this respect, these latter practices are scarcely contrary to phenomenological (existentialist/humanistic) orientations to therapy— with their strong emphasis on individual conscious agency (Fowers and Richardson, 1996; Martin and Sugarman,1999, Spinelli, 1995). And in this same regard, the differences between these orientations and cognitive therapy begin to whither. From Kellyian constructivism to mainstream cognitive therapy of today, the critical concern was—and is—with the individual's construal or cognitions of the world (see, for example, Mahoney, 1995; Hoyt, 1994; Rosen and Kuehlwein,1996). More specifically focused on the shared meanings within the culture, and the use of therapy to reconstruct these meanings is a host of more recent therapeutic practices. Here I would include a range of narrative therapies (White and Epston, 1990; Goncalves, 1995), brief therapies (DeShazer, 1994; O'Hanlon, 1993), postmodern therapies (Anderson, 1997; Riikonen and Smith 1997), reflecting teams (Anderson, 1995), social therapy (Newman and Holzman, 1999), and a range of more linguistically oriented systemic therapies (Hoffman, 2002; Tomm, 200; Griffith and Griffith, 1992; Friedman, 1993; Penn and Frankfurt, 1994).

With respect to engendering skills of resilience, I fear we are only at the beginning. So much attention has been given to talk alone, that attention to other forms of action has been neglected. Most promising at present is the development of meditation skills, a form of action that can furnish relief from the intense stresses of daily life. Much needed, however, are means of enhancing skills in conflict reduction, detoxing personal failure, avoiding over-commitment, acting collaboratively, and moving improvisationally across complex contexts. Traditions of cultural life furnish numerous avenues to suffering; the challenge is to develop resources for moving through cultural life effectively as opposed to sedating ourselves for the journey.

Research: Nothing About Us Without Us

Virtually all mental health research, treatment practices and policy formation is in the hands of professionals. While reasonable in many respects, it is also to say that decisions affecting the lives of millions of people—often in dramatic ways—are made by a small number of people, few of whom have ever experienced the problems they confront, or have themselves lived with a diagnoses of "mentally ill." In effect, those who have the most extensive and intimate experience with suffering, therapy, and pharmaceuticals, have virtually no voice in the decisions affecting their lives.

In the area of human disability there has been a lively resistance movement. Those labeled "disabled" find the ways in which they have been defined, segregated, and dismissed highly abusive. James Charlton (1998) provides a glimpse into the emerging passions:

> The dehumanization of people with disabilities through language...has a profound influence on consciousness. They, like other oppressed peoples, are constantly told by the dominant culture what they cannot do and what their place is in society. The fact that most oppressed people accept their place (read: oppression) is not hard to comprehend when we consider all the ideological powers at work...In the case of disability, domination is organized and reproduced principally by a circuitry of power and ideology that constantly amplifies in the normality of domination and compresses difference into classification norms (through symbols and categories) of superiority and normality against inferiority and abnormality. (pgs. 35-36)

This movement among the disabled is now developing with rapidity among those who feel variously abused by current mental health practices. The anti-psychiatry movement of the 1960s has new wind in its sails. Both regional and world-wide movements of ex-mental patients have now sprung to life.[1] Numerous academic journals and international conferences give scholarly voice to these issues. In effect, we are witnessing the formation of two combatant camps – the majority of mental health professionals on the one side and those who feel abused by the system on the other. Meaningful dialogue is rare. In my view it is incumbent on the mental health professions to instigate just such dialogue. Those who are affected by the profession should be systematically included in developing research policies and practices, in evaluating therapeutic procedures, and generating more promising pharmaceutical treatment.

In Conclusion

The preceding remarks represent a critical confrontation with the burgeoning movement toward understanding and treating problems traditionally understood as "psychological" from a neurobiological standpoint. I have first outlined a number of major costs incurred by presuming the neurobiological bases of human problems. I have touched on the spiraling and costly trajectory of "cultural drugging," the emerging myopia with respect to the cultural context of human suffering, the dehumanization of treatment forms, and the deterioration in value centered deliberation about our cultural future. I have turned attention to the rapidly expanding domain of brain research, which research has provided strong support for the neurobiological movement. Here we confronted important problems inhering in the isolation of relevant brain states, strong potentials for brain responsivity to cultural conditions, cultural biases in the interpretation of brain state data, and the ultimate inability of neuroscience to account for meaningful behavior.

Given the immense costs of the neurobiological orientation and the problematic grounds on which it rests, I put forward three proposals for slowing the current momentum and opening broad deliberation on a more promising future. My specific concerns were with imposing restrictions on the prescription of pharmacological treatment, prioritizing treatment forms specifically engaged in transforming cultural meaning, and opening up dialogue on issues of "mental illness" to those most intimately acquainted with such problems.

In the end, however, I must admit to a certain degree of skepticism regarding the future. The pharmaceutical industry has enormous wealth and a highly effective organization. The power of the pharmaceutical lobbies almost insures there will be no governmental intervention. And too, the managed care industry has thus far proved more invested in profitable outcomes for itself than grappling with the complex challenges confronted here. Further, the insurance companies profit by reducing coverage for "talking cures." Finally, the psychiatric profession stands to gain financially by the current trend, and prescribing drugs provides a certain degree of security against malpractice litigation. Therapists from outside the medical profession—clinical psychologists, social workers, family therapists, counseling psychologists, nurses, and the like—have largely buckled under the demands of the insurance companies for psychiatric diagnosis. At present I cannot recognize any important source of organized resistance.

In the preceding chapter I advocated litigation as a means of removing the demand for psychiatric diagnosis. In my view the single most powerful lever of change may be legal. There is one significant point of vulnerability in the current rage toward pharmacological treatment. Psychiatrists are essentially using a disease model of diagnosis, and prescribing medication with virtually no evidence of a neurobiological malfunction. The side effects of these prescriptions—both biological and psychological—along with the disinterest in terminating prescription are injurious to clients. Increasingly we learn of clients whose suicide can be traced to pharmacological treatments. As discussed in the preceding chapter, there is an increasing number of ex-patients—from around the world—generating organized resistance to the ways in which they have been diagnosed, treated and culturally defined. Perhaps it is in the "return of the repressed" that class action litigation will take route. I would count this as a victory for human well-being.

Part III

Explorations In Relational Flow

6

The Poetics Of Psychotherapy

A poem should not mean
But be.

Archibald MacLeish

If we hold that human communication is a matter of one mind registering the state of another mind, we would never communicate. Rather, as proposed in Chapter 1, let us understand communication as a process of human coordination. In this sense we may even say that spoken and written language represents the most highly nuanced, sophisticated, and multi-potentialed means of coordination available for the development of relationships, culture, and viable society. It is through language (both verbal and non-verbal) that we come to be constructed as individual selves, endowed with qualities, and evaluated as good or bad. Or more broadly, all that we come to hold as reality, as possessing value, as worthy of continued life finds its roots within our jointly created forms of language. To escape the "house of language," in Heidegger's terms, would be to exit relationship, culture, and meaning. There is no clearing outside in which we might deliberate, for outside relational process there simply is nothing *for us*.

As we see from these preliminary remarks, language can itself be constructed in many ways, as a *house*, as *coordination*, as *meaning*. With each characterization we also open new vistas of understanding, and thus new possibilities for action. This fact has profound implications for the therapeutic venture. As proposed in previous chapters, therapy is primarily an excursion in meaning, a process of human coordination by which past, present and future are constructed and reconstructed. And it is the hope and promise of this process that somehow, out of the swirling concatenation of meanings, possibilities for a new life will take shape. Yet, this "somehow" deserves our continuing attention; never can we be certain precisely where and how the door was opened—if at all—to an altered (and from some standpoint, "better") mode of being. For what we make of therapeutic process is itself a byproduct of our conjoint process of making meaning. Thus, we are perhaps best served by opening the therapeutic process to a multiplicity of characterizations, with each new lens lending itself to new sensibilities, and forms of practice.

It is in this vein that I wish to take up what can be called the *poetic form* of language. In speaking of poetic language, we typically call attention to rarefied and highly valued qualities. Let me focus on three of these: When we speak of language as poetic we are often referring to its *unsettling capacities*—to the ways in which we are moved, absorbed, or aroused. It is the rare juxtaposition of words and phrases that seems to pierce the veil of the ordinary, and move us into different dimensions of understanding. Second, we speak of language as poetic when it gives *credibility to the imaginary*—placing wings on whimsy, or bringing fantasy to life. Poetic language takes license to exit the ordinary and invite us into worlds of wishes and wonder. Finally, we speak of the poetic when language brings forth a *sense of the aesthetic*—arresting us with its beautiful symmetries, mellifluous harmonies, or enchanting rhythms. It is in the poetic that we somehow transcend the rag-tag and often brutish juxtapositions of everyday conversation to achieve a sense of the sublime.

With these three qualities of the poetic dimension in focus—the catalytic, the imaginative, and the aesthetic—we may address the central question of this chapter. If therapy is an excursion into meaning, how can we animate its poetic dimensions? Do we not often hope that the therapeutic experience will unseat the common habits of mind and action with which the client enters, challenge the imagination in such a way that new wellsprings of motivation may be unleashed, and enable the client to live in ways that are more fully in harmony with the world? How can the metaphor of poetry, then, bring into the foreground aspects of therapeutic process that might otherwise go unseen? What would it mean for us as therapists—or as participants in our daily relations—to achieve the poetic in our relationships?

To explore these questions it will first be helpful to address some common suppositions about poetry. As I will propose, we will be benefited as therapists by shaking loose some of the traditional ideas about poetry and considering newly emerging conceptions of the craft. With poetry thus reconceptualized, we shall be positioned to return to the ways in which the poetic dimension can be realized within therapeutic practice.

Poetry in a Postmodern Key

We may define poetry in many ways, and this choice will largely determine what will be offered up in the way of resources for therapeutic practice. In my view the conception of poetry that that we inherit from preceding generations is badly flawed. Broadly speaking the traditional assumptions spring from the cultural context of 19th century romanticism and 20th century modernism. Required in the present case is a reconstruction of these assumptions in terms of postmodern/social constructionist ideas. The traditional assumptions with which I am chiefly concerned may be termed *individualist*, *mechanist*, and *rhetorical*.

The individualist supposition is that poetry represents the outpouring of the poet's mind (emotions, intellect, feelings, spirit, soul, etc.). Here we hold that the poet is one whose special sensibilities, keen perceptions, or charged imagination, enable him/her to create the poetic work. In short, the poet is the originary source of the poem. Consider the problems posed by this particular view of poetry for the therapeutic relationship. In particular, a therapist functioning in the poetic dimension is cast as a special sort of person, prized let us say, for his/her capacity to craft words that are unsettling, imaginative, or beautiful. It is the therapist whose depth, passions, or sensitivities give wing to the poetic. The client, in contrast, is reduced to the role of bland, and passive audience. He or she may applaud, be moved, appreciate or be awed. However, the result of conceptualizing the therapist as poet essentially favors a hierarchy in which the client occupies the inferior position.

This problem is intensified with we consider the individualist invitation to see the poet/therapist as an independent actor, the font of inspiration, somehow different from, superior to, and free of the surrounding society. As often characterized, the poet is speaking with his/her own creative voice; he or she is a lone visionary. By implication, the client is invited to identify and emulate, to locate the poetic within him/herself. The task is to tap into one's own creative energies, and realize the independent self—ironically, by following the therapist's example. In this way, therapy serves to foster a world of isolated, self-sufficient, self-important individuals. Relationships are not only secondary, but even suspicious, for they may inhibit or suppress the creative impulses.

There is an alternative to this view of the poet that emerges from postmodern/constructionist dialogues. As contemporary literary theory—from Barthes to Derrida—has made clear, an author is never an independent, originary source. Poetry only becomes so by virtue of its existence within a tradition of poetic writing. It acquires its intelligibility as poetry because of its resemblance to works within this tradition. If I were to call this chapter a poem, and submit it to a poetry journal, it would most surely be rejected. It would be rejected primarily because it fails to look or feel like poetry; it doesn't speak in the traditional voice of poetry. In effect, the poet never escapes relationship, but rather, owes his/her very existence as a poet to participation in relationship.

This dependence of intelligibility on relationship is simultaneously a hallmark of social constructionist theory. As we have seen, for the constructionist language only achieves its meaning within relational activity. Alone, one is deprived of the capacity to mean; truly private words would fail to communicate. In this context the therapist's actions must be viewed as deeply embedded within a complex array of traditions, traditions that furnishes most of the major resources for participating in the process of making meaning within therapy. The therapist's language is not rendered superior as a result of the therapeutic tradition; such language only acquires its capacity to mean by virtue of the client's assenting participation. Simultaneously, we come to value not the client's isolation from others (clothed in the raiment of "self-sufficiency"), but his/her active engagement in processes of meaning making.

Consider next the mechanistic presumption informing our present-day understandings of poetry. Here it is presumed that the poet's work *has effects* on the audience. The good poem will move its audience, cause them to see or feel things differently, or reveal to them profundities of which they were previously ignorant. In effect, the poem operates within a mechanistic system of cause and effect. Essentially such an account reproduces the mechanistic model of medicine that gave birth to the institution of psychotherapy. Here the therapist is the doctor who acts upon the patient to bring about cure. In parallel, the poet/therapist acts upon and produces change in the client. Yet, we have become much aware in recent decades of the problematic implications of the mechanistic orientation. It is not only that the client's knowledge tends to be discredited ("lacking in expertise") on this account, but the therapist is thrust into the role of manipulative strategist, objectifying and experimenting with the "object of study" (the client). Worse still, the therapist's private views of "the good" are little open to question, mystified as they are by the neutral, expert language of "cure." In the hands of experts, for example, a child's impetuous curiosity can be "poetically" transformed into Attention Deficit Disorder, with no questions asked. After all, the therapist is the expert, and can act upon the child to bring about cure.

Again, in the domain of poetry, postmodern literary theory serves to challenges the mechanistic view of poetry and literature, and thereby opens new vistas. In particular, literary theorists call attention to the role of "the active audience" or "the interpretive community" in determining the meaning of a work. Rather than a poem or literary work *acting on* an audience, it is reasoned, audiences play an active part in determining how the work is interpreted. "Reader response theory," as it is called, demonstrates the multiple and indeterminate array of meanings that may be attributed to a given literary or poetic work, depending on the interests, values, ideology and the like of the reader. There is no "poem in itself." Poetry is given birth in a relationship. As outlined in Chapter 1, this is also a line of argument congenial to much constructionist dialogue. As reasoned in this case, meaning is not the possession of single minds, and communicated with efficacy (or not) through words. Rather, meaning is always generated within relationship, within the process of mutual coordination.

Finally, we inherit a conception of poetry that is rhetorical. That is, from Longinus to the present, we have presumed that the potential of the poem to create effects lies in its particular arrangement of words. Certain words or phrases—in contrast to others—have the capacity to create beauty, passion, pathos, humor and so on. In effect, the poet is a rhetor, whose power over the audience depends on his/her linguistic craftsmanship. Yet, when the rhetorical metaphor is extended to the therapeutic domain we also find reason to resist. Within this metaphor it is again the therapist who is granted the power—through language—to effect changes in the client. The client is merely an object to be transformed through the rhetorical artistry of the therapist. Most case studies in therapy are indeed analyzed in just this way, with the strong emphasis placed on the way in which the therapist crafts his/her words to create the desired effects. By the same token, we seldom see how it is that the clients' words have functioned (craftily?) so as to give the therapist license for his/her contribution. In effect, the client is denied status as an effective rhetor.

From a postmodern/constructionist standpoint, words in themselves have no power. This much should have been made clear in the preceding comments. Rather, for the constructionist the "power of words" derives from their function within an ongoing relationship. Consider the case of "sustained eye contact." Under many circumstances such an action is noxious: "he is always staring at me," "I feel like I'm being cross-examined," "I wonder what the hell he is thinking," are all possible responses. However, when inserted into a candlelight conversation, replete with hints of romance, "sustained eye contact" becomes "a significant gaze" and its power more intense than any words. Poetry, like eye contact, acquires its rhetorical efficacy not from its particular arrangement of words and phrases, but from the way in which it is embedded within relational space.

Therapy in the Poetic Dimension

Our analysis of the poetic dimension has placed a strong emphasis on catalytic unsettling, imagination, and aesthetics. As I have argued, however, if we accept the traditional view of poetry—in its individualist, mechanist and rhetorical mold—working in a poetic dimension has a range of unfortunate consequences. We sustain traditions of power, manipulation, and separation within the therapeutic relationship. However, if we reconfigure the conception of poetry along postmodern /constructionist lines, we can nurture the poetic dimension in different ways and with different outcomes. In this case, we locate the poetic dimension within relationships as opposed to individuals, and the focus is on meaning and movement through coordinated action. We are drawn to the possibilities for mutually negotiated meaning, and the significance of words and action within particular relational contexts. Poetry, on this account, cannot be created either by you or me, but grows from the relational process. We realize the poetic dimension together.

Yet, this account remains all too abstract. In what manner might therapeutic practices achieve the poetic? Informed by a social constructionist sensibility, how can therapy engage in the poetic processes of *unsettling the ordinary, stimulating the imaginary*, and enhancing a *sense of the aesthetic*? In my view many existing practices make a substantial contribution poetic realization. However, their major achievements fall within the first two domains; it is in the realization of the aesthetic that we find the primary challenge for the future.

Unsettling the Ordinary

Consider first the unsettling or catalytic aspects of poetry. If our sense of the real and the good—and thus our sense of joy, anger, depression, and the like—are generated within relationships, then we may view any "problem" reported by the client as the residue of past relationships. "My awful life" is the result of *some form* of relationship. The poetic challenge is thus to enter into a relationship that can unsettle the existing stasis, and soften the ground for developing alternative realities—ways of understanding self and others otherwise obscured by the "obvious truth of awfulness." Of course, the use of therapy to unsettle the ordinary is scarcely new. Indeed from Freud to contemporary cognitive therapy, practitioners have sought means of challenging the everyday understandings of their clients. However, with the increasing consciousness of the ways in which our worlds are constructed in language, the concern with language as a "dithering device" has become focal. In this sense, the systemic development of "circular questioning," the narrative focus on "restorying," and the multiplication of stories via reflecting teams (Anderson, 1991) are excellent entries into the poetic vocabulary.

However, I have been especially taken with practices stimulating multiple voices within the individual. The Western tradition has long placed a value on the singular self—a unified, authentic, and coherent core self. It is this vision of the singular self that is largely responsible for our defining multiple personality as a "disorder." and our labeling certain patterns of puzzling behavior as "schizophrenic." This same emphasis on the singular self has also functioned as a barrier to exploration of the multiplicity of being, the possibilities that we carry with us at any time multiple and often conflicting potentials. Inconsistency, vacillation, incoherence, ambivalence—all such terms carry with them negative connotations. It is in this light that we can appreciate the importance of practices that enable clients to explore their multiplicities. For example, Karl Tomm's (1998) exploration of multiple "internal others," and Penn and Frankfurt's (1994) process of multiple letter writing, both create new and important conversational spaces. It is also in the opening of multiple voices that the dimensions of relational being become more apparent.

Creating the Imaginary

Let us turn to the second aspect of the poetic dimension, namely the emphasis on stimulating the imagination. How is the imaginary to be nurtured within the constructionist conception of the poetic? In some degree we grapple with the challenge of the imaginary in attempting to unsettle the sedimented realities with which clients enter therapy. Any conversation that moves into new spaces of meaning will necessarily be a stimulus to the imagination. However, the problem of the imaginary has yet another dimension. It is not simply an unfreezing of the settled that is at stake, but the generation of a discourse of desire, that is, a discourse that creates images of a future that nurtures hope, excites, and entices.

In my view it is this exploration of the imaginary to which therapies congenial with constructionism have made an especially significant contribution. Traditional therapies are backward looking. Therapists ask for recountings of the past, why did you feel that way, who did what to whom, what precipitated the current condition, and the like. In effect, therapies that search for origins, trajectories, structures, and dynamics create the reality of the past. It is this reality that may come to dominate the conversational space of therapy. In contrast, a constructionist consciousness invites a focus on future realities—visions of a livable world, positive possibilities, and viable outcomes. It is this creation of a positive vision that provides direction and hope. Solution focused therapy (O'Hanlon and Wiener Davis, 1989), and its replacement of problem oriented discourse with solution talk, is an obvious case in point. In brief therapy, "the miracle question," (deShazer, 1994) also shifts the conversational reality in the direction of an imagined future. Drawing from the day to day vernacular, resource oriented therapists move toward a positive conceptions of the future. O'Hanlon's more recent work (1999, Bertolino and O'Hanlon, 2001) places a special emphasis on positive possibilities. My colleagues at the Taos Institute, David Cooperrider and Diana Whitney, work more broadly with a process called *appreciative inquiry* (see www.taosinstitute.net). Here talk of problems is suspended, and participants recount positive incidents (narratives) from the past. However, with these narrative resources in hand they embark on discussions of how to create a future together. All such practices are poetic creations of the imaginary.

Fostering Aesthetics: Orders of Challenge

Finally, how can the therapeutic relationship nurture the aesthetic dimension of the poetic? How can relationships move toward the sense of beauty? There can be no single answer to this question, as there can be no single standard or criterion of the aesthetic. From a constructionist standpoint the very idea of beauty is a construction of a culture, and its standards may evolve with time and circumstance. And so it is within daily relationships. We generate criteria of the beautiful—which may tend toward simplicity or complexity, repetition or novelty, etc. There are many ways of achieving a sense of the aesthetic in daily relationships.

At the same time, we may ask: are there not certain processes of relationship necessary to create any form of the aesthetic? What is it about a relationship that grants the very possibility of beauty? If we can identify such processes can we not say they constitute a primal aesthetic source?

Without this primal source beauty becomes an impossibility. Inquiry into transformative dialogue (Gergen, Gergen and Barrett, 2002)—points to a number of dialogic moves that seem essential in the present case. Two of these are well represented within existing therapeutic practices. The first is *affirmation*. As proposed in Chapter 1, in order for any utterance to acquire meaning, another must provide some form of affirmation. Another must supplement it in a way that it comes into meaning. Failure to acknowledge someone's words, or negating them ("No, that isn't right...") puts their meaning to death. Required for realizing the aesthetic are actions that do not suppress and negate, but give birth to meaning.

A second important means of realizing the aesthetic is through *dialogic metonomy*. Metonomy refers to the use of a fragment to stand for a whole of which it is a part. Thus, "the golden arches" are used to signify the McDonald's restaurants, or the British flag to indicate the United Kingdom. Dialogic metonymic occurs when one's actions contain some fragment of the other's actions, a piece that represents the whole. If I express to you doubts about my parents' love for me, and you respond by asking, "What's the weather report for tomorrow?" you have failed to include my being in your reply. Dialogic metonomy is lacking. If your response includes the sense of what I have said, possibly concern over my doubts, then I find myself in you; I locate in you the "me" who has just spoken. At the same time, because it is you who have generated this expression, it is not quite mine. You move us closer, and in doing so, I am invited to reply metonomically to you. Metonomy is achieved in the therapeutic relationship in the therapist's simple acts of responding to the client in ways that reflect or incorporate the client's preceding words.

Many clients leave the therapeutic hour with a sense they have experienced a special form of relationship, in certain respects ideal in its degree of openness, understanding, and caring. In effect, one may say that they have experienced the primal creation of an aesthetic. They have entered relationships in which the therapist has affirmed their utterances and responded to them in their terms (more commonly we might say, the therapist has "listened well.") Yet, most therapists face a far more challenging task, one for which adequate resources are not yet available. Many people enter therapy precisely because they exist in relationships in which the primal grounds for the aesthetic are absent or seem impossible to achieve. Consider a relationship in which mutual negation dominates: you can say nothing that I find agreeable, and all that you favor I find annoying. There is little in such a relationship that will nourish the development of an aesthetic. Beauty will never come into being.

Let me call this the *second order challenge* of restoring the aesthetic. The first order exists when there are no grounds for mutual animosity or negation. This challenge, is easily achieved within most existing therapies. Good supportive discourse comes close to the mark. The second order challenge is far more difficult. Relationships of mutual negation are common fare in the world outside therapy; within the therapeutic hour they are almost non-existent. More importantly, the skills manifest and available for modeling in the first order relationship of therapy are of little value in the more common condition of second order challenges. I cannot easily apply skills of affirming and reflecting in a hostile relationship. If someone is verbally assailing me, it is very difficult to nod in assent. To be sure, the therapist may help the client to "understand his or her condition." But understanding is a description from outside. That is, the words we use here and now to "understand my situation" are not frequently those I use in "doing my situation" there and then. A newly discovered narrative of myself as "survivor," for example, is not something I may easily place in motion in my daily conversations. Required is usable discourse adequate to the second order challenge of restoring the aesthetic.

In my view family therapists are in the most optimal position to articulate and make available such discourses. This is so because the process of mutual hostility is often brought into the consultation room. It is there before us. Explanation from the outside may be offered, but more importantly, new forms of discourse may be encouraged, new moves in the conversation suggested and put into practice. There is now a great need for these practices to be articulated and shared. It is the "knowing how" of restoring the aesthetic that needs to be made manifest. In our work, Relational Responsibility, Sheila McNamee and I tried to take an initial step in this direction. Our concern was with the mutual hostilities set in motion by individual blame—accusations of wrong-doing—breaking a rule, irresponsibility, misjudgment, callousness, stupidity and the like. So often we respond to such accusations with irritation, and when we do we often enter into a continuing scenario of mutual hostility—or "the blame game." Our attempt was to develop an alternative vocabulary, one that would enable participants to step out of the common scenario and restore the possibility of the aesthetic. We treated, for example, the conversational use of multiple voices, relational explanations, inter-group explanations, and references to the larger context. All can be used to restore more affirmative relations. Yet, this exploration is only a beginning. Locating and/or creating a vocabulary of relational restoration may be viewed as a primary challenge for the future.

7

From Treatment To Dialogue: Reflexive Cooperation In Theory And Practice

With Eugene K. Epstein

Many therapists now view the construction of meaning as central both to the creation of individual and family problems, and to the process of therapeutic change. It is in this vein that narrative therapists view clients' narratives as central to the creation of "the problem," and re-storying as the major means of moving forward (Epston and White, 1992; McLeod, 1999). Brief therapists shift attention away from the "reality of the presenting problem," to exploring future possibilities, visions, or scenarios (de Shazer, 1996 ; O'Hanlon & Rowan, 1999). In the work of Anderson and Goolishian (1992 a, b) a major emphasis is placed on the systems of meanings in which the individual or family is enmeshed, and the kinds of client therapist relationship that allow for the emergence of new meanings. All such ventures owe a debt, as well, to the Milan systemic therapists and their concern with the shared and reiterative logics of the family (Boscolo et al, 1988). As Hoffman (2002) recently pointed out, Gregory Bateson's early emphasis on communication as the basis of psychiatric change "was the seed of the flower to come." (Bateson & Ruesch, 1951, pg. 259)

Yet, in spite of this increased focus on the social construction of meaning, many important questions remain unaddressed. For one, families involved in the therapeutic processes do not generally describe such encounters as those of equal participants searching together for possible meanings and solutions to human dilemmas. They instead tend to describe such interactions as being rather difficult, if not conflictual interchanges amongst unequal partners (Epstein 1992). How, then, are new and useful realities to be generated in therapy when there significant power imbalances exist within a family? (Pakman, 2000; Hoffan, 2002). Closely coupled with this problem is the challenge of conflicting realities. How is one to work successfully with client systems in which various members hold divergent, competing or perhaps even incongruent goals? Must one choose sides? And how are we to respond to clients who have ideas that are very different, if not diametrically opposed to the therapist's? Do we need to convince our clients of the superiority of our professional views or should we suppress our own opinions in deference to the clients?[1]

From a theoretical and practical standpoint such issues are of pivotal importance. Constructionist theory emphasizes the importance of the co-construction of realities, rationalities and values. When there is an unequal distribution of power, such that certain participants have little voice in the construction process, the stage is set for resentment and conflict. This is but one of many viable explanations for what today are commonly called "psychosomatic" and "psychosocial problems." Those denied voice may be mobilized to create alternative realities, to resist what appears as the arbitrary and misguided world of the superior, and subtly set out to undermine the dominant discourse. Under conditions of unequal power, then, how can parties be brought into synchrony?

Closely related is the challenge of antagonistic realities. Commitment to a given construction of the world often carries with it disregard or disrespect of those who do not share or agree. When such constructions are suffused with a sense of "good" and "right," those failing to share may become contemptuous. Simply understanding what those "on the other side" believe is insufficient to reduce the gulf of separation. From within one's world, such beliefs are obviously erroneous or ominous.

Again, the question is raised, how can one proceed to bring conflicting parties into a new and more inclusive perspective? Questions such as this are crucial to building a fully mature conception of therapy as social construction (Gergen, 2001).

On the practical side, issues of power and multiple realities are particularly important in therapeutic work with adolescents. Power differences are virtually endemic within the family, but the adolescent period is often one in which the voices of authority are thrown into question. Here too, the adolescent often has the support of his or her peer group in creating alternative and perhaps resistant realities. And too, spousal differences in power are not uncommon, as well as the triangulation of one parent and child against the other parent. The gulf separating participants within the family can be both extreme and intense. Practically speaking, then, how are these conflicting and power based conflicts in reality to be brought into a viable relationship?

It is typical within the therapeutic profession to generate answers from within the profession itself. We take it upon ourselves to fashion both the legitimate questions and the possible answers regarding effective therapy. While such a view is warranted in terms of both the depth of experience and continued reflection, there are also limits. Chief among them are the lived worlds of our clients. From a constructionist standpoint, we take seriously the view that psychotherapy is most effective when the clients themselves actively participate in defining and re-defining their lives, determining their goals, proposing their own solutions and are actively engaged with the therapist in the process of change. It is this emphasis on processes of co-construction that also begins to point the way toward solving the dilemmas outlined above. As professionals we need not—and should not—proceed independent of our clients. Our clients' futures should not be enshrined before they ever enter the door. In what follows, then, we offer an approach to the above issues that allows us to bring important resources into the therapy room that may enable progress to be made without a priori determining its particular trajectory.

Toward a Theory of Reflexive Cooperation

In thinking through these questions we have come to develop a conception of reflexive cooperation, and to explore its potentials within the therapeutic setting (Epstein et al 1998). To appreciate what is at stake it is first useful to examine some of the more common ways of understanding the term "cooperation." One of the more prevalent views of cooperation sees it as a set of techniques for achieving compliance, such as in "medical compliance." This idea of cooperation implies that the so-called "good" patient will acquiesce to the better knowledge of the medical expert as to how to improve his/her health and/or well-being. The patient abdicates thinking about and evaluating among various conceptions of health and well-being, and is expected to carry out recommendations provided by the expert. Absent from this form of exchange is the recognition that notions of health and well-being are socially constructed and not god-given, or universal (Epstein, 1992).

Another common understanding of cooperation equates it with consensus-building. It is not hard to think of examples in which dominant voices and discourses have suppressed or silenced alternative voices (See Levin et al 1998; Hoffman, 2002; Weingarten, 2003). This is the very danger we see in confusing cooperation with consensus. In contrast to these conceptions of cooperation, we favor a view in which all parties set out to work with each other toward a common good. This is not to seek a singular or dominant discourse, an ultimate set of agreements about the real or the good. Rather it is to honor the differences and to ensure that participation is open to all. In principle, cooperative discourse should have no fixed point of termination, no line beyond which no further voice can speak. In effect, cooperation becomes an ethical stance in which we are ultimately responsible for the process of relationship itself (McNamee and Gergen, 1999).

To this conception of cooperation we add reflexivity. We also attach special meaning to this term. By reflexivity we do not mean the process of turning back to reflect upon one's own position or utterances. When one's utterances construct a given world of the real, rational and good, reflections on such utterances will essentially recapitulate the same set of understandings. Reflections on any system of understanding from within its own premises will never enable one to transcend the limits of the system. In our view, reflexivity establishes the need for deliberating on a given construction of the world from multiple, diverging standpoints.

In our view, reflexive cooperation is indeed an ethical stance; but it is far more. When people share discourses of the real, rational and the good, they also share forms of life. Such forms of life often offer security, nurturance, and a rationale for action. To dismiss or silence a given discourse is to threaten a tradition dear to the participants. The results are divisive, and ultimately invite the very kinds of schisms now destroying thousands, if not millions of lives across the globe. In contrast, when given forms of life can be opened without threat to alternatives, new possibilities emerge, new sensitivities can develop, and new amalgams can be generated. It is this kind of "edgework" that enables sharp differences to be replaced by common and creative concern. (See also Gergen, 2002.)

In the therapeutic context we propose that there are no transcendentally superior or expert discourses, per se, that is, discourses that have a more accurate, objective, or discerning grasp of what health and well-being are or indeed of how to achieve them. Rather different discourses, emerging out of different traditions, open up particular possibilities, or more specifically, open up new relational possibilities while excluding and disallowing none. The usefulness of any one discourse can only be determined locally, by the participants themselves, in terms of the possibilities they offer in light of the goals and values they hold. It is our opinion that reflexive cooperation must allow divergent voices to emerge, especially those that have been marginalized. And this is a particularly urgent imperative within psychiatric interactions in which the dangers of dominant professional discourses silencing the voices of clients are manifold (Gergen, 1994).

In our vision reflexive cooperation is a process through which the relationally generative elements of reflecting teams (Andersen, 1990, 1997) are first extended across the spectrum of therapeutic interchanges. Not only would this apply to relations of therapist to family, and among family members themselves, but as well to the broader community that forms the vital context of family well-being. Ideally we would wish to see processes of reflexive cooperation extend to the mental health professions themselves. The community of practice should be vitally enriched, with current schisms and conflict giving way to mutual and respectful collaboration. Here reflexive cooperation joins hands with existing ideas of the shared power of definition, tolerance for incommensurate ideas, solidarity or multi-partiality, constructive feedback, and curiosity. We understand these terms as building blocks towards more inclusive futures.

Reflexive Cooperation in Action

Ideas such as these are more effectively appraised in terms of practical consequences. In practice, we believe that it is well worth the effort to actively invite clients and their families to define with us together the expectations and goals for our conversations together. Questions regarding who should participate in conversations as well as in which constellations, the frequency of such meetings, the question as to whether the conversations shall occur on an outpatient or inpatient basis, the possible topics or questions to be discussed, as well as what shall not be discussed or when the conversations should no longer be continued, are all decided jointly. In this sense, we no longer speak about therapy as "treatment" but rather as a dialogical process, the conjoint development of old and new possible narratives. Here we offer two illustrations of reflexive coopera-tion in practice:

A Boy's Freedom: The Case of Parent/School Conflict

The teachers of an 8 year old boy met together over concern for their pupil. They were seriously concerned over the parenting abilities of his mother. Though their efforts a crisis meeting was convened. It consisted of helpers and helping family members (including teachers, child protec-tive services [Jugendamt], adult psychiatric outreach social workers [Sozialpsychiatrischer Dienst], the mother's brother, the mother and one of the authors [E.E.]). The mother had suffered a psychotic episode just prior to becoming certified as a grade school teacher many years before and had never worked outside the home. She was partially physically disabled as well and walked with a severe limp. Shortly after having her first and only baby, her brother had visited and discovered that the child's father had long since deserted her and that she and the child were living in very isolated, unhygienic, and life-threatening surroundings. The brother arranged for his sister and nephew to move in next door to him, where he could help take care of both.

At the beginning of the consultation, there was uncertainty and much hesitance among those present about just how to begin discussing the multiple concerns about the mother's ability to parent adequately. In pre-vious talks between the teachers and the mother, the teachers had tried to persuade the mother to allow her son more freedom and independence. She walked him to and from school everyday, often bringing him into the classroom itself, in violation of the teacher's expressed wish that the mother no longer enter the school building. They had learned from the boy that he was not allowed to visit with other children after school or go to the playground on his own. The teachers believed that the mother of-ten did the boy's homework for him and were told that she would force him instead to take two to three hour naps each afternoon. The mother talked often about her son's "medical condition" which necessitated his not being allowed to run around or overstress himself physically. The boy's uncle had also tried without success on numerous occasions to convince his sister to grant the boy more freedom of movement. The mother had responded with anger and the threat to move out of the area with her son, as well as a threat to write letters to the school board calling into question the teachers' competency.

As the meeting began and the various helpers began to talk about their concerns for the boy, the mother talked over the others and animatedly defended her position. After a few short minutes, the consultant questioned all present as to the apparent difficulty in agreeing to how we might all be able to talk as well as listen to one another. All agreed that this was not yet possible. The question was then raised as to how the conversation might proceed such that all might get a chance to speak and be heard. After a pregnant pause, it was the mother who spoke up. She suggested that the professionals just talk among themselves, not speaking to her directly so that she might listen without feeling compelled to immediately defend herself.

As the professionals began to talk about their concerns, the mother started to take notes. After a time, she suggested that a contract be drawn up among all present. As she explained it at a later meeting, she would be more readily able to grant her son more freedom when she had more of a sense that she was being supported in this effort from others around her. The contract, as well as her suggestion about how to talk together constituted creative offerings for a more cooperative conversation. All participants agreed to a follow-up meeting several months later to evaluate the changes at that time.

In the ensuing weeks, the boy began making contact with other children he would meet at the local playground and no longer had to visit his uncle in secret. The teachers were relieved that the mother was no longer writing complaints about them to the school authorities and pleased that the boy was now doing his own homework and walking to and from school by himself. The mother was relieved that she was not being held responsible for her son's development in and out of the school, and slowly gave up doing her son's homework for him. The therapist was relieved that this mother, who was initially being described as incompetent and indeed harmful for her son's development, was now being described more positively. The danger that this child and mother might be separated from each other against both of their wills (a possibility that had been discussed more than once by the authorities) had lessened greatly.

Was the process of cooperative reflexivity perfected in this case? This is a question that opens a new round of reflexivity. From our perspective, distinct improvements would be made by having the son more directly involved in determining his future. The difficulties of encouraging this young boy's voice among so many competing adult voices, is not to be underestimated. How much pressure might he feel to remain loyal to his mother? To his teachers? His Uncle? How would this affect his ability to speak freely? How did he view the conditions, the relationships, and the potentials? Further, it would have been useful to establish a means of continuing the process of deliberation. All agreements are achieved under conditions at the moment, but the contingencies of daily life are forever in motion. In any case, by inviting the "designated patient" to contribute to the outcome, a creative and effective move was facilitated.

A Girl's Fear: A Case of Parent/Child Conflict

Close to a year ago, a fourteen year old girl. Julia, was brought to a meeting with one of the authors (E.E.) accompanied by her foster mother and the supervisor of the foster mother. Julia had been living for almost a year in the foster family, after authorities (das Jugendamt) had decided to separate her from her mother, stepfather and siblings. The separation was to protect her from her stepfather, against whom allegations of physical abuse had been made. Julia was described as suffering from encopresis and enuresis as well as aggressivity and difficulties getting along with peers and adults. The situation in the foster family was described as very difficult and the foster mother reported that Julia frequently abused her verbally. Julia was also doing poorly at school and was in conflict with her teachers and fellow students on a regular basis. At the age of ten, while she was still living with her family, she had been hospitalized for several months in another child psychiatry unit with similar presenting problems.

The foster mother, the supervisor and indeed Julia herself had discussed the idea of hospitalization among themselves prior to our meeting. All were in agreement that Julia should be hospitalized. The therapist spent time slowly and carefully discussing everyone's ideas and wishes surrounding a repeat hospitalization. The therapist opened a reflection on why they all thought that another hospitalization would be helpful when the first hospitalization did not seem to have been so. Within this conversation the therapist also asked Julia for her ideas about how she could envision discussing the hospitalization with her mother. The mother still had legal custody and would therefore be required to grant her permission for the treatment.

Julia at first replied that her mother had nothing to do with the therapy or her life at this point and should therefore not be included in the decision. When the therapist asked for her advice about how they might deal with the mother if she requested information (as is her legal right), Julia became very angry and walked out of the room. After a time, the foster mother went out to speak with her and soon they both re-entered the room. The therapist apologized to Julia for upsetting her and remarked that the mother seemed to be a rather difficult topic to discuss. Julia agreed about that and we all agreed to meet again and think about how to find a way to talk about the "problem of mother" with each other that would be acceptable for all.

In several meetings that followed, we began to reflect on how to speak with each other about the mother so that Julia would not become upset. As we were exploring various ways to do this, we then began to think about having Julia's mother join in the talks. We also had to consider possible dangers. Julia's biggest fear was that if we talked with the mother, we would believe what she said and then stop believing what she had told us. She described the mother as a liar and someone who could not be trusted. She recounted that when she had told the mother about being hit by the stepfather, her mother had initially supported her and helped her file charges against him. Later the mother had dropped the charges without telling her. Julia accused the mother of remaining loyal to the stepfather even though he had beaten her as well as the children, and she worried that her younger siblings were also in danger.

As our talks progressed, it became apparent that all of us, including Julia, could talk about the mother's participation. By this point Julia had said that the very difficult and complicated relationship with her mother was a very important. if not central issue, for her therapy. Much time was taken discussing all of the possible ways the mother might decline an invitation to meet, as well as the many options about how one might best invite her. Finally, Julia herself offered to call her mother and invite her personally.

The mother did respond positively to the call and several conjoint meetings were held. At first Julia confronted her mother with accusatory questions. Her mother failed to attend the next meeting and told the therapist on the telephone that she was not happy with the meeting. She felt that she was under investigation and had little chance to explain herself. She did finally agree to attend further meetings, but mentioned that her work schedule, as well as her many responsibilities at home for her three younger children made planning difficult. As we continued to meet, Julia tried to explain to her mother why she "hates" her stepfather. The mother admitted finding it hard to believe all that her daughter was telling her, but made it clear that it was indeed her wish to continue trying to understand her.

The sessions continue as of this writing. In the meantime, Julia, the foster mother and the supervisor have all agreed that hospitalization at this point is no longer necessary and have asked to remove Julia's name from the waiting list for admission. The foster mother related that she and Julia now got along much better, that Julia is doing much better in school and that the enuresis and encopresis have all but disappeared. Julia is no longer fearful that the stepfather might suddenly emerge to threaten her; instead she talks about inviting him to participate in our talks as well. Julia's mother is also encouraged that she is now beginning to talk differently with her daughter. She no longer feels cut off from her daughter, but instead actively engaged in thinking through her future. Many issues remain open in the case and the future is far from determined, but the conversations continue.

Toward a Vocabulary of Reflexive Cooperation

The preceding cases are especially important in demonstrating the power of those in therapy to make important contributions to their future well-being. In the initial case, it is the designated patient herself who creates an option that will lead to major improvements—for her son, her son's teachers and friends, and ultimately for herself. In the second case, again we find the suggestions of the "problematic" adolescent to be pivotal in directing the course of subsequent conversation. It is she who ultimately invites her mother, long the object of intense distrust, into the therapeutic conversation. The results broke the lock of a dysfunctional relationship. At the same time, it must be realized that these contributions are not spontaneous. That is, they emerge from a specific form of conversational process. Required is the cooperation of the therapist, at a minimum, and in

both the present cases of others relevant to the case. Further, these cooperative activities have certain characteristics which facilitate the kinds of
reflections that engender change.

Let us consider these characteristics in terms of *discursive vocabularies*. That is, by using language in particular ways, the therapist (and
other participants) contribute to reflexive cooperation. Because it is not
possible to lay out in advance the trajectory of conversation, it is impossible to specify precisely what discursive entries will be productive at any
given time. Rather, it is more profitable to think in terms of a vocabulary
of discursive moves from which the therapist and others may draw selec-
tively. In the cases described above we would identify the following elements of such a vocabulary:

- Respecting the client's constructions of the world. It is perhaps to
  Carl Rogers (1951) that we owe the significance of this orientation
  to the client's accounts of self and world. However, this orientation
  is now prevalent across the range of meaning centered therapies.
- Requesting opinions on fruitful courses of action. The emphasis
  on the client's ideas for fruitful action has featured importantly in
  resource or possibility oriented therapies (O'Hanlon & Rowan,
  1999). Here it becomes the center-piece of reflexive cooperation.
- Avoiding unilateral, authority based decisions. Coupled with inquiry into others' views on fruitful ways to proceed, the cooperatively centered therapist avoids making unilateral, authority based
  decisions. In this way, reflexive cooperation is strongly influenced
  by Anderson and Goolishian's (1992a, b) views on "not knowing."
- Broadening the circle of participation. In both the cases above, a
  strong emphasis was placed on inclusion. As reasoned, for reflexive cooperation to be effective, it is important to have the participation of as many people as possible who are invested in the outcomes of therapy. In this way, reflexive cooperation owes a debt to

Tom Andersen's (1997) emphasis on expanding the range of relevant intelligibilities. As well, reflexive cooperation resonates with the work of Jaco Seikkula (1995, 1996) on dialogic teams.

- Focusing on relationship. In reflexive cooperation a strong emphasis is placed on exploring dimensions of relationship. This stands in contrast to many therapies concerned primarily with the private psychological life of the client. In our view, whatever is private originates in patterns of relationship, past and present. Therefore, it is to the relational matrix that primary attention must be directed.

- Avoiding person blame. Closely related to the preceding, reflexive cooperation is more effective when the therapist and others avoid conversations in which individual blame or censor is likely to result. In the initial case above, care was taken not to allow the mother to take the blame for what seemed her wretched treatment of her son. In the second case, it was critical to diminish Julia's anger toward her mother.

- Emphasizing affirmation as opposed to censor. Also resonating with the avoidance of blame is the strong use of affirmation in therapeutic work. Many suggestions may be offered by participants in the therapeutic process, and the therapist may often feel such offerings are misguided or even injurious. However, it is typically useful to affirm the potential wisdom of all offerings, regardless of private thoughts. Typically, in the process of inquiry other, more promising options will emerge, and these can be supported more enthusiastically. The use of censor or criticism will often remove the participant from the cooperative process.

- Reflecting on the participatory process. At crucial junctures it is important to turn the process of reflection back on the process of cooperative reflection itself. As in the case of Julia, for example, it was important at one point to have our own ways of talking become the subject of reflection. Because the communication process within the group is pivotal to the outcome, this process may require periodic attention.

These eight discursive options have played a central role in our attempts to bring the concept of reflexive cooperation into effective practice. When and where they are effectively insinuated into the therapeutic conversation cannot be specified in advance. Significant experience might be necessary for one to "get the feel" of when and how things can be said. At the same time, we do not see these options as exclusive. They form the grounds of what we hope will become a far more extended vocabulary. Indeed, we trust that our clients will take part in generating still further possibilities for effective cooperation.

8

Exploring The Terrain: From The Personal To The Professional

Mony Elkaïm interviews Kenneth Gergen

Mony Elkaïm is the Director of the L'Institut de la famille et des systems humains, *in Brussels, a consultant in the Department of Psychiatry of the L'Hopital Erasme, and the past President of the European Family Therapy Association. Elkaim is the author of* If You Love Me, Don't Love Me *(1989) and* Panorama of Family Therapies *(1995).*

M. Elkaïm: We might begin by having you briefly introduce yourself by telling us about your background. Then we can explore more fully some of your ideas and the relationship to psychotherapy.

K. Gergen: From whence do I come? Just how should I describe this to a therapist? Let's say that professionally, I was trained in experimental social psychology, a very empirically oriented, systematic, disciplined study of human social behavior. Over time, however, I became disillusioned with the hopes and aspirations of this field. Somehow I felt there were fundamental problems in making sense of my own life in terms of the theories and methods of the discipline. I also became very concerned with the transient quality of much of the phenomena we were studying. The discipline took pride in drawing from its work universal conclusions about thought, emotions, motivation and so on. And yet, all the phenomena under study were here today and gone tomorrow. Worse still, as we began to describe and explain these phenomena, the descriptions and explanations themselves became forces within society that altered the very patterns that we were attempting to describe. I formulated these and other doubts as a series of critiques, which led to an enormous amount of controversy at the time. My work contributed to what became known as "the crisis in social psychology."

M. Elkaïm: When was that?

K. Gergen: This was in the mid-seventies. I wasn't alone in my concerns and I certainly must also credit some of the self-reflexive critique to the ambient political ferment of the time. For us, it was the Vietnam war period; there was enormous social unrest, and a broad questioning of the political agenda that seemed hidden under the claims to neutrality in science. So I was joined in the critical posture by many scholars from different sectors of the profession—ranging from existential humanists to Marxists. The result for me was a separation from the traditional mainstream of the field and an entry into discussions with philosophers, sociologists, anthropologists, a number of others who were worrying about the future of the human sciences. I became very concerned with trying to formulate a way of thinking about human science which was more livable, more practical, more humane, more impassioned and more promising in its potential for the society. I can say a lot more about those issues, but in brief my concerns led over time to the development of an alternative way of thinking about ourselves and the human sciences. This development was over ten years in the making, and has now coalesced in a movement called social constructionism. In the constructionist view, all that we take to be real and good is an outcome of human relationship, both in science and everyday life.

M. Elkaïm: Can I ask you a little question here? Your position on that point seems quite close to Maturana's. Is there a difference in your positions on that particular point?

K. Gergen: Well, for me it depends on what part of Maturana you read. If you look at early Maturana and the sort of frog's eye view of the world, I think it's quite different.

M. Elkaïm: I'm referring to the fact that for Maturana, for example, he speaks about objectivity in brackets, the fact that two researchers can speak about their research without in fact having to deal with reality but only with their own constructions.

K. Gergen: Social constructionism does share with Maturana a conception of "reality in brackets." However, the way in which you arrive at this conclusion is quite different. This difference is also very important in terms of implications for therapy. His questioning of objectivity is, again, primarily through that early research on the frog's eye where he wants to say that we each create in our own brain, you might say, a conception of reality. Thus any production or any representation, any statement about the real, is a by-product of the individual's own particular standpoint or structural determination.

M. Elkaïm: I think there is more to it if you allow me, because I wasn't thinking so much about his work on the frog's eye, but about when he began to work with human beings and to study the perception of colors. The interesting thing is that you cannot obtain from objective sources the link between what's happening in the brain and the color: it is in language that these things appear. So there he's speaking about the link between perception and language.

K. Gergen: Again, Maturana begins here with an individualist presumption, in this case the perception or understanding of the single individual of an independent reality. If you begin with this presumption you confront the epistemological problem of how the internal mind can ever reflect the external world. To solve the problem he must add a social or linguistic dimension to the account. The individual must acquire language as a means of understanding color; in this sense the individual must take on the social as a supplement to the personal. The social constructionist orientation is a quite different in the sense that it begins with the social; it begins with relatedness and not within the single individual. The entire epistemological problem—how the external becomes internal—is bracketed as well; it, too, is a problem created in language.

M. Elkaïm: This is very important. Can you say a bit more about that?

K. Gergen: Philosophically speaking, if you privilege the reality of the individual minds (or subjectivity) as your starting place, it is very difficult (I think impossible) to solve the perrenial problems of philosophy, for example, how external reality is accurately represented in the mind, how we understand other minds, or how we generate comprehensible language. In spite of 2,000 years of philosophy, these problems have never been adequately solved. For example, you can't simply start with, let's say, a blank slate (Lockian) view of the mind and ever explain how the individual acquires language. Chomsky has demonstrated this quite clearly. However, if you posit a set of a priori conceptions (an innate knowledge of language) as do Kant and Chomsky, you find that the individual can never learn anything that is not already built into the pre-programming. If I'm programmed to understand the difference between black and white, I can't derive green from this a priori distinction. I've written a fair amount about these problems in my book, Realities and Relationships.

M. Elkaïm: So let's now come back to the way you created your own theory.

K. Gergen: I can't really claim to be the origin of my work, you see, because all intelligible theories could only come into being through relationships, through some form of dialogue. Even the intelligibility of "I" is a sensibility created through relationships. This is an important point, so let me say a little more. As we coordinate ourselves with each other, out of the coordination may come various distinctions like "I" and "you," along with "my experience," "your intention," "your emotions" or "my thinking." In effect, the very language of comprehending individual minds is a by-product of relatedness. It is not individuals who work together to create relationships, but it is to relations that we owe the very sense of being individuals. So the ontology, the epistemology and the ideology of social constructionism are quite different than for the constructivist.

M. Elkaïm: What you are saying is very important, because for a lot of us, it was that realization, that you cannot speak about an individual as separate from his context, which created the field of family therapy. What you are saying is that nothing appears in the mind of the individual just like that, it appears in the context of the relationship he is in. So please continue, and try to describe your work and how you think it is affecting the field of psychotherapy and family therapy.

K. Gergen: Yes. When we place our central focus on relatedness, and the way in which relatedness generates meaning and the sense of the self, we are speaking very directly to issues in family therapy. It seems to me that the original significance of family therapy was derived from its contrast with individual therapy; it promised to break away from the narrow focus on individual mental events. Over time, however, individualism crept back into the vernacular, for example, in the view of the individual as a self-organizing system. In many ways I see social constructionism as offering family therapists an alternative set of metaphors, you might say, or vehicles for reflecting on the process of therapy itself. Constructionism moves away from the family of mechanistic metaphors—the cybernetics, servomechanisms and feedback loops—that once dominated the field. It also offers alternatives to the physicalistic or biological metaphors , and as well the cognitive orientation that treats the social world as a kind of a secondary byproduct of individual minds. So to me, as I've talked with many therapists, I find constructionism offers a rich family of concepts, a challenge to the idea of human "deficit," new openings to productive practices, and a different view of the therapist's role. Because social constructionism is born out of wide-ranging discussions taking place in literary theory, symbolic anthropology, feminist studies, post-modern anthropology, discourse analysis, and the like, it provides an entry into a new set of discussions for many therapist.

M. Elkaïm: Before going further, could you just summarize for me and for our readers how you define the terms modern and post-modern?

K. Gergen: You ask questions which one really needs an entire day to answer!

M. Elkaïm: I know, but there are so many definitions.

K. Gergen: That's right; the discussions do seem endless. For purposes of this conversation, however, let's look at look at modernism as a world view, an overarching ideology, and a set of related cultural practices which largely derived from guiding metaphors within 16th-17th century western thought. The tendency was (and still is) to view the cosmos as one large machine, that is, as composed of elements systematically related to another. The individual, in the modernist view, possess the capacity to observe and to rationally comprehend that machine, and thus to generate increasingly accurate knowledge of the cosmos. With the increased capacity for prediction and control, we may anticipate unlimited progress. So there's a great emphasis on mechanistics, the sanctity of individual minds, objectivity, rationality, and progress. This view informs most all our major institutions since the Enlightenment, including government, education, law, and so on.

M. Elkaïm: So you would put Marxism and Hegelianism in modernism.

K. Gergen: Marx and Hegel did share in the idea of history as moving in a progressive direction; and Marx's belief that there is a single, rational system of economics that can be imposed on a society is clearly modernist. The belief in broad governmental and city planning, universal principles of art and architecture, and the importance of scientific (rational, objective) thought in everyday life, are also modernist in the way I am using the term here.

M. Elkaïm: And then post-modernism for you is...

K. Gergen: For many it begins with the modernism turning on itself to question its own foundations, and finding these improbable or impossible. Now that's too simple a view historically. If you return to the 1960-70s and all the political ferment, they can be seen as the return of a romanticist anguish over the moral emptiness of modernism. The emphasis on objectivity, rationality and progress seemed to subvert any kind of moral sensibility or commitment. So within the political eruptions, you find an anger with modernist establishments—government, business, science, the military—that had seemingly no moral foundations, no special telos other than to acquire increasing abilities to control or gain greater power for themselves.

M. Elkaïm: So you could see, for example, in post-modernism a demand for ethics?

K. Gergen: In the early stages I think that was one of the stimulants. I think this precipitated a wide range of self-questioning, but since then the dialogue has moved on dramatically. This continued reassessment of foundations, of purposes and so on has turned now even to question the possibility of ethics and political meaning. I think it is also crucial to our understanding of postmodernism to attend to the vast effects of our communication technologies—the media, the computer, the telephone, and the like—which rapidly saturate us with new and contrasting intelligibilities. As I discussed in my book, The Saturated Self, the result of this enormous immersion is a sense of relativism, of multiple goods, multiple rationalities. This too has been a significant influence on the postmodern temperament.

M. Elkaïm: So how would you define today a post-modernist attitude in relationship to science, to politics, to everyday life?

K. Gergen: Again, I think you'd have to be highly differentiated as to which particular group you were talking about, but let me talk a little about social constructionism because that's very much part of this dialogue.

M. Elkaïm: With pleasure.

K. Gergen: If you look to the intellectual world, there's been one great wave of despairing critique of modernism for the last ten to twenty years, a vast deconstruction of the modernist hopes for rationality, objectivity, progress and so on. In my view, social constructionism offers a means of escaping the despair, a more positive opening to new forms of thought and practices. That is, constructionism is a movement that takes advantage of the critique but isn't simply its repetition. Its view of rationality, objectivity, of ethics and so on would be to say that, yes, within a subculture, within a special ethos, you can generate a sense of the objective, the real, and the good which is very compelling and to a degree very useful; within a subculture such as science you can develop theories which come to have the sense of being truly objective, truly accurate. However, it is essential that these views be treated as artifacts of these local processes of relating as opposed to universals.

This is where the "Maturana brackets" are relevant: all realities must be placed in brackets as a means of avoiding the calamities resulting from the tendency of communities to treat their realities as necessary and good for themselves on all occasions, and necessary and good for all peoples everywhere. In this sense constructionism removes the nihilism of many postmodern writings. It recognizes the essential need for the sense of objectivity, rationality, and the good. We must not excuse ourselves for our traditions, for without them there should not be a world-for-us. We don't abandon everything that lacks foundations, but rather, recognize the limitations. And we see that our traditions are located within a world of alternative, competing, and contradictory realities with which conciliation is essential. One of the major challenges we now face is how then to go on together in a world of saturated selves—a world which, by virtue of technology, is making that set of competing realities clash with ever increasing frequency. This is so all the way from the world of the family therapist to international policy making, and it is a problem that requires yet new constructions of self and other.

M. Elkaïm: My dear Ken, can you describe, and I apologize for the didactic aspect of the question, some of the specific points of the theory you developed in the context of your peers and over all these years which you think could be useful for the field of psychotherapy and for family therapy in particular?

K. Gergen: With pleasure. I think it's important here, however, to understand the sense in which I mean theory and how it could be useful. As a constructionist I say, "Don't take my theoretical musings as a reflection of the truth; rather, these ideas are resources for our conversations, for our ways of going on together; the issue is not their truth but of our well-being—humanity's well-being as we use these resources." So I am not proposing a theory that therapists can then apply straight away, but trying to engage in conversations that may have productive potential within the communities within which we live.

With this said, constructionism first suggests that in therapy we do not approach the client with a strong or routinized set of suppositions and methods, such as those often associated with psychoanalytic, behavioral and cognitive theories. Therapists' theories are themselves constructions, and in this sense can operate as blinders. Here I find much value in the Goolishian-Anderson orientation to therapy of "not knowing." Second, as therapists, it is important to see the client's narrative, not as reflecting the true nature of the problem, but as a contingent construction. We try, then, to understand language, not as a reflection of the real, so much as a pragmatic device, that is, a mode of relating in itself. So if the client speaks of despair, dire problems, or depression, for example, that language is not descriptive of a real depression or a dire problem, but reveals a way of relating to others, with certain kinds of effects. You might say the construction invites certain kinds of dances; it precludes others.

Third, we take the emphasis off subjectivity—the emotions, thoughts, repressions and so on—of the individual client; we remove the exploration of the interior of the client as a major concern. Rather, we shift the focus to the client's context of relationship, and begin to explore the pragmatic significance of the client's narratives within these contexts. With whom and for whom do they make meaning; if these are the accepted narratives within these relationships, what follows for the client and others? This also means approaching conflict in terms of competing constructions (not as issues requiring adjudication according to some universal criterion of the true and the good.) Modes of negotiation are required that enable meanings to be coordinated.

As you can also see, for the constructionist there is also a strong emphasis on the therapeutic transformation of narratives. Are there alternative means of comprehending the self and others, modes of discourse that will play out more effectively in the range of existing and potential relations? Here I like to place a special emphasis on multiple narratives. The point is not to replace one fixed but defective story with another fixed mode of understanding, but to help the client to take advantage of language or sense making as a rich resource for living with others. In a complex social world, the capacity to shift and transform realities is essential. In a sense, one must ultimately transcend narrative. This also means recognizing—and I think you very much share this idea—your own contribution to the generation of meaning in the therapeutic setting, your role as co-constructor of the real and the good.

M. Elkaïm: Earlier you mentioned your book, "The Saturated Self." When was it published?

K. Gergen: In 1991 by Basic Books. It would be a pleasure to send you a copy.

M. Elkaïm: I also have to send you a copy of "If you love me, don't love me," which was published by Basic Books in 1990. You will see how I move away from the world of systems at equilibrium by first criticizing the systemic approach through Prigogine, then entering the field of second cybernetics, still remaining close to Heinz von Foerster's position, but already beginning to create a lot of elements which go completely in your direction. For example, the tools I created are tools which enable us to think about our feelings or our constructions as psychotherapists or as supervisors in the context where they emerge. You no longer think about something which has to do with some kind of projection, like in the old way psychoanalysis would look at that, or as counter-transference, but as something which emerges in the social context created not only by the family in therapy and yourself, but also by other systems, or other contexts which are in intersection with that situation. These contexts can be, for example, the institution where you see the patient, the supervision group or the social rules of the context in which you find yourself. By the way, I started by calling that situation an "intersection" until Heinz von Foerster told me, "Call it a 'resonance', it's more dynamic," and I think he was right. It is interesting to see that reflecting on the self-referential paradox of the psychotherapist who is drawing a map of a territory in which he finds himself led me to a situation where I couldn't think any longer in terms of an individual boundary, but of something emerging in a context. From that perspective, feelings are no longer feelings which originate only in myself. That is perhaps where they seem to appear, but they are emerging in a specific context of social interaction.

K. Gergen: I see many ways in which we converge, different vocabularies and different emphases but in the same conversation.

M. Elkaïm: Some of the people in French-speaking countries have heard about you through, I would say, a limited knowledge of the work of people like Harry Goolishian or Harlene Anderson. For example, when some of the practitioners in French speaking countries hear a sentence like, "We want to dissolve the problem in conversation" or, "There are no functions, no meanings," then they think, "How can we work? How can we make sense of the behavior of someone if we don't have any hypotheses?" The interesting thing is that, for me for example, it's important not to know what is good for people. This situation or position of perplexity is important, but at the same time, something has to emerge in the context of the work with the people to enable them to be relieved of their predicaments, or at least live their predicaments in another way, with less pain.

K. Gergen: I had been very close to Harry before his death and to the work he was carrying on at the time. I do think that when you write or speak you often look for some simple and dramatic ways of putting things, ways that are easy to grasp. However, the result is often overstatement, and thus unfortunately of resistance.

M. Elkaïm: I'm going to put this interview side by side with an interview with Harlene Anderson where she explains her ideas in more detail, and where the reader will be able to see that it's a lot more complex, a lot richer than they think it is when they listen to some kind of slogan.

K. Gergen: I think that's a nice idea. Harlene's work is very much a contribution to the constructionist dialogues in therapy.

M. Elkaïm: Can you try to define social constructionism?

K. Gergen: Let's look at social constructionism as a set of conversations which are taking place around the world on the communal genesis of meaning, understanding, knowledge, and value. These conversations call into question all our taken for granted assumptions, all claims to authoritative knowledge, and all that we have taken to be essential about the self. At the same time, they invite us to see ourselves as inherently interdependent, and to see that our future depends not only on how we manage these interdependencies, but on our capacities for communal transformations in our constructions of self and world. I must add that these conversations don't attempt to fix precisely the nature of constructionism, to canonize it so that it's owned or guarded by anyone. However, there is general sense of an enormous liberation and accompanying excitement in the vast potentials—intellectual, political, cultural, and indeed global.

M. Elkaïm: Is there something else you would like to add, Ken?

K. Gergen: Well, I could go in several directions here. But let me say a little more about self and culture, and especially about multiple selves and the possibility for one's existing in multiple realities simultaneously. We emerge from a modernist tradition which honors the unitary coherence of the private individual. That is, we hold that one's thoughts should be consistent, one's feelings should not be contradictory, one should not be divided against the self. The self should strive toward singular identity, in Erikson's terms. From the constructionist perspective, however, we are not independent of our relations. To have a self at all is to be related. And, if our relationships are multiple, with differing opinions, values, and feelings generated in different contexts, then the idea of a unitary self becomes counterproductive. To demand coherence or singularity is to ask for an ineffectual mode of being. It's as if we borrowed from the Platonic conception of ideal mind, instituted it in our educational systems, and ultimately constructed it as the ideal personality. Perhaps in a world where close knit and continuous communities were modal, such a conception was viable. However, in the saturated world of the postmodern, it is virtually inconceivable. Further, when we remove the yoke of coherence from our individual lives, we find vast relief—an invitation to move with the ocean of relationships in all its multi-directedness.

M. Elkaïm: This is fascinating, because some of my work with a French psychoanalyst called Felix Guattari, who wrote a book with Gilles Deleuze entitled, "The Anti-Oedipus" and another one called "A Thousand Plateaux," focused on a point very close to that. For example, you will see in my book, "If you love me, don't love me" a discussion about how, in Proust's book, "Remembrance of Things Past," Swann falls in love with Odette. It's not a case of an individual who falls in love, it's what I call an "assemblage," a number of different elements jostling to get into relation. For example, when Swann looks at Odette for the first time in the Verdurins' salon, he doesn't find her that attractive. However, there's someone playing music, and there's the fact that she looks like Zipporah, the daughter of Jethro, in a painting by Botticelli in the Sistine Chapel in Rome. He buys a reproduction of that painting to put on his table. And there are a lot of little elements which add to each other, and this kind of assemblage—Guattari would call that an "agencement" in French or an "arrangement" in English—is going to create that change in him: he falls in love. My friend Guattari always had a problem with family therapy and he would constantly say to me, "How can you speak about individuals and relationships? What does the 'individual' mean?" He thought more in terms of "arrangements," and I myself used to speak of systems of assemblages rather than systems of individuals. In fact, that part of my work is used very little in the field of family therapy because it seems very difficult, rather than speaking about systems of individual relationships, to speak about the interrelationship of elements which are completely diverse: they could be genetic, organic, of a mass media nature, as well as something relating to a specific piece of music. I don't know if that's close to what you're speaking about.

K. Gergen: Yes, wonderful. I love this notion of the assemblage. It's a striking metaphor that can set us in motion in many different ways.

M. Elkaïm: I took the notion of assemblage from the surrealists. For example, the simplest assemblage is that of Picasso, who took a bicycle handlebar and a saddle, put one on top of the other, and called it a bull's head. Obviously, there is nothing of a bull there, but still for everyone it's clear. This is the most simple assemblage: two pieces are juxtaposed and something new appears.

K. Gergen: Marvelous. But why not extend the idea of the assemblage to see the person's parts as also assembled together with parts of others? In this sense, I am not an assemblage unto myself, but all the parts assembled in the being before you are embedded within still other assemblages. To put it another way, I see myself in this conversation as only an illusion of an individual. Yes something we call "I" is speaking, but what you don't see and what is of enormous significance in understanding this "I" is the vast range of relationships which are now manifest here, which are never specifically identified, which I represent but do no re-present.

M. Elkaïm: What work do you use generally? Do you use multiple voices?

K. Gergen: I do find the metaphor of multiple voices has a lot of currency just now. I like the connection it makes to various other works, particularly to literary theory and especially Bakhtin, and to feminist theory and the salient work of Carol Gilligan. The metaphor carries a rich history.

M. Elkaïm: Peggy Penn uses that a lot also.

K. Gergen: Yes, Peggy Penn has been very much part of the constructionist conversations. For therapy, which is largely a voicing process, it's an easy metaphor to take on. More importantly, it is richly suggestive. It suggests that for any voice the client presents to you, he or she probably harbors many others, each of which could carry the conversation in another direction, and some of which could even negate what is currently being said. It draws attention always to the possibility that whatever is being said could be something else, that there is not a unified self operating here, that you could set in motion another voice in that conversation where the person could deconstruct or at least put limits on the world as he or she is currently constructing it. Whatever is seen as a tragedy could be a comedy if you allow the others to speak, whatever is hostile could be loving if you allow the voices entry into the conversation. By the way, here is an illustration of the way theory becomes important not because it tells the truth, but because it provokes reconsideration of practices. For

Peggy, I think, the metaphor has very much been an invitation to her use of letter writing in therapy. In asking the person to write various sorts of letters to various important others, she is giving them an opening to other voices embedded within other relationships.

M. Elkaïm: Could you say a little more here about the role of the therapist?

K. Gergen: There is much to say, but let me link this to the earlier discussion of multiple communities, and multiple realities in a globalizing world. At this point I see the definition of the therapist as a specialist in healing "the ill"—the definition we inherit from the medical tradition, as terribly limiting. For the constructionist, the therapist doesn't stand outside society; therapeutic work essentially builds society, politically, ideologically, morally. Thus, why confine our skills as co-constructors to individuals and families? I think this expansion in awareness is slowly taking place (even if it is sometimes stimulated by the economic situation). For example, I have been working with a number of family therapists who are trying to expand their practice into the realm of organizational development. They find that many of the skills in coordinating meaning within families are highly effective in the organizational setting—businesses, non-profit organizations and government. There's a therapeutic institute in Cambridge, Massachusetts which has made itself available to the United Nations to aid in otherwise conflict ridden discussions of population control. They have been very effective in coordinating these discussions. As I mentioned earlier, we now face a global situation where the multiple realities of various groups are coming into increasing conflict. It seems to me that there is a vital opportunity developing here for family therapists to reconstitute the profession—to see its implications and potentials in far more sweeping terms. Can therapists, who are daily immersed in the challenges of coordinating meaning, also serve the society in cases of more searing conflict among groups—political, ideological, religious, and so on? Can we rise above specific partisan commitments to generate means of communication or coordination among otherwise competing groups which will allow us to live more easily in the world together? There's a tremendous challenge here.

M. Elkaïm: That's interesting. I just wrote an article for a journal called the Palestine-Israel Journal, which is a journal published by Palestinians close to Arafat and Israelis fighting for Israeli-Palestinian coexistence. They asked me to write an article in an issue on the psychological implications of the conflict, and I used my model of couple therapy to speak about the Arab-Israeli conflict, showing how conflict appears not only in the couple, but also in the context where that couple exists, and how if we link what is happening at the level of each of the participants to the people around them or the nations around them, we can start thinking in a different way.

K. Gergen: This is an excellent example of how we might being to apply more systemic thinking to more global political issues. The next question would be, what kinds of practices could we offer if we were party to these conversations?

M. Elkaïm: In my case, it led me to create in the seventies, with Jean-Paul Sartre, something we called the Israeli-Palestine committees, which were difficult to accept for the majority of people: for a lot of Arabs, we were Zionists because we were defending Israel's right to exist, while for a lot of Israelis, we were anti-Israeli, because we were defending the right of the Palestinians to have a state. We created these committees at the end of the sixties, and today the coexistence of two states is the official position of the Palestinians, and will soon be that of the Israeli government, when it accepts that there will be a Palestinian state alongside an Israeli state. So perhaps dialogues have more chances of survival than discussions about who is right and who is wrong.

K. Gergen: Yes, exactly. And then the question is, what sorts of dialogues would they be and how can we facilitate them? These are not practices that can be derived from a theory; they must be hammered out of daily experiences in working with others. Theory may help to articulate, share, and stimulate. However, there is no replacement of the hands-on skills developed in daily relationships with clients.

M. Elkaïm: Exactly. You're totally right because the way those committees came about was that I myself was very involved in the student movement in the sixties and, by chance, I happened to be in the right place at the right time, I played an important role in the student movement in Brussels. Lots of my friends were completely pro-Palestinian, against the existence of Israel, and lots of my other friends were pro-Israeli, and all of them were in the same left-wing group, all struggling for a better society. It was interesting for me, in a situation where I had friends on both sides, to try to create a dialogue between them. It was not created solely because I am a Moroccan Jew who was raised as a Jew in the context of an Arab culture that I loved, that helped me perhaps in the right social context to be able to be part of a bridge, but if there wasn't that particular social context, those committees would never have existed. Once the committees existed, then something could begin to happen. So your question about how we can create dialogues is interesting, and this is quite complex, but I like your idea of multiple voices, because in all of us, at some moments, some voices for dialogue, for openness, for hope are completely silent. We don't even know we have them.

K. Gergen: To continue this concern with dialogue, one of our inherited traditions for settling conflict is that of logical argument. Here is a resource ready at hand, almost reflexively taken for granted by many people, and yet so ill equipped for today's problems of difference. In argumentation the opponents attempt to demonstrate the superiority of their view over the other. It's a combat model in which each side attempts to vanquish the other. I treat you as having a unified logic, and if there is any incoherence in your logic, I immediately use it to destroy you. Now if we take that tradition of argumentation as our form of dialogue, there's no way in which our contemporary problems—Arab/Jew, pro-life/pro-choice, Western/Islamic fundamentalism, and so on—are going to be alleviated. Based on our experiences in coordinating diverse realities, we must develop other forms.

M. Elkaïm: The problem for me is this: suppose that you are open, that you are trying to maintain an openness in relation to me, and suppose I see every sign of openness of yours as something which means that I'm the one who is right. The tragedy is that you are putting yourself in a situation where you are in danger because I'm not going to enter into your dialogue. My whole logic and the context in which I find myself are such that everything you do, every step you make towards me is taken as proof that I am right. When we touch on some of these aspects in psychotherapy, luckily for us it's not dramatic, because in psychotherapy, if a patient is continually attacking me, and I refuse to become defensive, after a while the patient begins to feel a new feeling in the relationship: "How come, although I'm attacking him all the time, he remains open?" Sometimes a patient will leave, because a social context is created in which he feels very uneasy, and as we would say, in our language, he prefers to maintain his armor and protect himself by leaving rather than open up. But often people will accept to open up and that situation of dialogue in psychotherapy is very rich. In effect, the psychotherapist will use himself in such a way that he will not accept to enter a dance of non-dialogue and he will help the others in the family to maintain a position of dialogue. It is more difficult in political life where a lot of interests are vested in a situation that is a lot more complex than psychotherapy or family therapy.

K. Gergen: Yes, it's as if we have as a therapeutic community managed to see the limits inherent in the traditional individualistic, or monologic approach, and now we begin to explore the potentials of dialogue. We find that argumentation as a dialogic form is deeply problematic, and begin to explore more cooperative means of interchange. Here we find ourselves confronting yet a new challenge, that of the "one reality" orientation. But again, we confront this problem in part because of the cooperative tradition we inherit. The task, then, is to experiment with still new alternatives. This is a privilege we have in the therapeutic encounter. We must focus on expanding the repertoire of capacities in therapy to include much more active exchanges—such as your idea of what I would call being a model, that is, offering another set of alternative actions where you don't, for example, reciprocate an attack with counter-attack, but demonstrate the possibility of a new relational form.

M. Elkaïm: It's not really being a model, but rather trying to play a different role in the social context which exists between that person and myself. I'm not trying to be a model, I'm trying not to be where he wants me to be, if what he wants me to be at that moment is something which will repeat the pattern. Obviously, that's what I'm thinking, perhaps I'm completely mistaken, perhaps that's the way I'm constructing it, but in that openness, there is the possibility of finding some common ground where something can be constructed, but I don't see myself as a model. If you want to use the old systemic terms, I would say that in the therapeutic system, I'm trying to avoid a situation in which the rules of my family of origin, of my context, and the rules of his context fall so in love with each other that they create some new rules which unite us in a process of repetition of our fears and our limits. Let me give you an example of this: once I was in New York in my car, and I was on the highway. There was a guy behind me honking, he was very, very upset, and he cuts in front of me and gets out of the car. So I got of my car and I said, "Listen, I must have been doing something terrible. I'm sorry, I didn't realize what I was doing." He was so flabbergasted, because he was coming to fight and honestly, I think he must have been right, because he was so upset, I must have been doing something I didn't know I was doing. Perhaps I was distracted, but I was so convinced by his anger that I could only say to him, "I'm sorry, I apologize, I didn't realize what I was doing, but I'm sure you're right." He left very uneasy! So I'm not trying to act as a model in that context, I'm just trying to maintain something open.

K. Gergen: There are many ways you can frame what you are doing. Another one that I like very much is in terms of the dance metaphor where I would see you taking the unanticipated or disruptive step in the traditional dance. You're violating the dance and therefore creating the possibility of a new dance form.

M. Elkaïm: I would say something different. I would say, when I come to psychotherapy and another person comes to psychotherapy, we're both bringing a lot of steps that we know. I never think that the therapist is swallowed, nor that the patient is swallowed: what we do is sculpt ourselves mutually in such a way that we create an apparently new dance, but it's a new dance with old steps.

K. Gergen: Which it must be, it must combine what we inherit from the past. A new assemblage of the relationship.

M. Elkaïm: And the art of psychotherapy lies in maintaining, on the one hand, an alliance around the dance while trying on the other hand to avoid steps which will lead to the same conclusions. And that's the art, I would say, of dialogues.

K. Gergen: I should add that one of my abiding concerns these days is in the capacity of the therapeutic conversation to carry over into the life of the client. Does the new dance transfer to anything else in the person's life? We run the risk, it seems to me, of creating a wonderful dance within the therapeutic setting, which works very well, and in which we have dislodged the previous rituals, but have generated a way of going on that is specific to the therapeutic context alone. There is the question of the extent to which our newly developed dance can be taken out of an office, and put into practice with people who are simply doing the other steps. Thought must be directed to ways of facilitating the exportation of the new resources.

M. Elkaïm: Suppose there is a female client who says to me, "I feel shitty. Either you are interested by me, in which case you're a shitty psychiatrist, and I don't need a shitty psychiatrist, or you're not shitty, so what are you doing with me?" And suppose that I say to her, "Well, I hear you, but I have no answer" and she will yell at me, "But I want an answer!" and I will say, "But I have none. I don't think I am shitty, and I don't think you're shitty, but I have to respect the fact that you feel shitty and that you are in that predicament. I respect it, I feel how difficult it is for you and I'm sorry I have no answer. I can only be on your side in that predicament and be part of it." If I do that, regularly, then something is going to happen in that context where she will begin to feel something about herself, about me, which is different. And that kind of dialogue, where I refuse to get in the position where she needs me to be, and where I help her not to get into the position where I need her to be in order to avoid reinforcing what I'm calling our world views, will help her, and me perhaps also, to walk differently in life, because what we learn in therapy will be used in life.

K. Gergen: Well, that's the question: can she walk differently? You've employed a very interesting, subtle, brilliant kind of maneuver that few others in her life will be capable of.

M. Elkaïm: Let's continue with this situation if you don't mind. For example, I take a plane, the plane arrives late and I miss the session. She'll see me next week and say to me, "I came for the appointment, I waited for you and you didn't come! And don't tell me you were on a plane, because at that moment, there were no planes!" This is incredible, I'm thinking, "How can she know that I was on a plane?" I'm not going to tell her I was on a plane, that would be defensive. I can only say, "I apologize, I was not there. I wanted to be there and I couldn't." And she'll say, "Where were you?!" and I'll say, "I'm sorry, I cannot get into that kind of exchange. What is important for me is that you were here and I wasn't, and I apologize for that. But getting into where I was and what happened, etc. is something which doesn't respect your feelings for what's happening." So after a number of sessions like that, she's going to give both of us more space. By the way, that lady was bulimic for years and years, with phobias, and the phobias disappeared, the bulimia disappeared, she got married, and she wrote to me saying "In the event that you played a role in me being better, I'm giving you some news." She left without being completely sure that I had been helpful. What I would say is, I created a situation with her where she could experience during the session with me, new ways of relating to someone else, she could free some new valances that she could use with others. I think you do that generally in various ways, for example, by giving tasks in the session, or at home. You do that in all the situations where something affective is happening at the same time as something intellectual, and sometimes there is no under-standing but there is something affective happening, and I think all psy-chotherapists can speak about that. Sometimes it happens during the ses-sion, sometimes outside of the session, and what we try to do is to create a context where people find themselves looking at others and themselves differently.

K. Gergen: I appreciate what you are saying, and most of the time I would not question it. However, we again inherit a tradition of therapy in which we trust that if we have "changed a person's mind"—let us say by giving them insights, or helping them to spaces of emotion—that their lives elsewhere will be bettered. But if we take seriously the assumption of multiple selves, assemblages, discursive relations, dances of meaning, and the like, it seems to me that we have to re-think this tradition. We must increasingly ask where and how these local conversations in the therapeutic hour can be exported into other practices. Let me expand on one aspect of this issue. Why should we limit ourselves to generating new alternatives, discourses, narratives and the like? These may be important, but why is it that we cannot actually share our perspectives, the languages that we use to describe and explain what we do? That is, you and I have no trouble talking about languages of dance, languages I would call mod-els, languages of assemblages and so on. That's important for us.

M. Elkaïm: I agree with you. In psychotherapy, we check the kinds of language of alliance we can have, and we find a way to connect according to the way people construct their world, without realizing it. This is why, for me, the first part of psychotherapy is crucial. It involves feeling how the others feel the world without being in their shoes. At the same time, we try to maintain some kind of space which will help them not only be understood, but also enable them to have a space of their own where they can construct differently.

K. Gergen: But to continue the question, you have an understanding of what you're doing which you feel is helpful because it's going to facilitate change. However, is there any way of communicating that understanding, so that they know what you know about relating? If we feel we benefit from our ways of talking about therapy, should we not share these languages with the client?

M. Elkaïm: This is very important. Your question is crucial. I think the way they learn is not through explaining to them what I don't know I'm doing myself. I don't know if the transmission of hypotheses helps people to change, I think it's more a case of a multiple assemblage made up of the dialogue around new hypotheses, of the affect which surrounds the exchange, of the sociocultural context in which it takes place, etc. Furthermore, my hypotheses are only operative constructions which are proposed to the family members to allow them to follow new paths.

K. Gergen: I totally agree that it is a construction of what you're doing, but somehow, for us in our community that construction is very important. I believe it makes a difference in our lives; I am sure it does in my own. We see the discourse as life-giving in some way. So when you construct yourself as resonating with the client's subjectivity, and feeling from that person's point of view, and trying to ask yourself how it is another would feel in relation, that very theoretical or reflexive move ought to have more of a place in the therapeutic conversation. I envision a world in which clients would be part of the set of professional interchanges. They would participate in professional meetings, and share in the activities of building our resources.

M. Elkaïm: I like what you're saying very much, and I have to think a little more about it. But I'm also thinking, how do I transmit to my students a way of being themselves? I believe that what creates something rich in psychotherapy is not only what we think we do, it's who we are. For example, when you see someone like Harlene Anderson in a session, the way she is, the way she smiles, the way she speaks, the clarity of the way she is, the openness, these are things that are very, very important and it's her, first and foremost, before being close to your point of view. So I think the interesting thing is also the marriage between who we are and our theory, and generally what we do is very simple. We choose the trainer, we choose the theory closest to our hearts, which makes it our theory and creates that blend which makes it so easy for us to behave in a way in which we blossom in that context. Of course, there are also people who don't choose, who find themselves with a trainer in a school and who, later in life, may choose a theory which is closer to their hearts than the one they learned first.

K. Gergen: I think something of that sort goes on, but imagine now taking our earlier discussion of multiple voices and expanding it to say to a client, "Well look, perhaps there's more than one me, more than one heart, more than one construction." Could this way of putting things not be exported from the therapeutic exchange?

M. Elkaïm: I agree completely with that. I think, like you, that we are multiple. And I think that not only are we multiple because we are divided into levels which very often contradict each other, but also we are multiple because different parts of ourselves can get into an assemblage with different elements of a context to create something different. For example, the same girl who is anorexic in her family will go to a friend's house and eat, or have less problems eating than when eating with her family. She's still the same. How come she behaves differently? You have a boy who is phobic in his family, he goes to boarding school and he isn't phobic. He comes home for the weekend and he's phobic again. So it's interesting to see that we have aspects of our personality which can ally with some context and get amplified in such a way that there will be a symptom. I like very much what you said about us being protean. I remember that R.D. Scott, an English psychiatrist working with Ronald D. Laing, once told me that there was a strike in a hospital and there was a guy who was catatonic, who didn't move. During the strike he was moving, doing things, and after the strike, he became catatonic again. It's interesting to see that guy had multiple possibilities and in one kind of context, a possibility became amplified and he behaved in one way, and in another context, he behaved differently. This is an aspect of your approach which I think is absolutely crucial, because it moves us away from the view of an individual as closed inside his or her skin and opens up the possibility of thinking in terms of what I call assemblages or interrelationships: part of us with part of the universe around us. Perhaps it is the relationship between assemblages which creates what we used to call a system.

K. Gergen: Let me offer a similar case to again keep this problem of exportation in focus. I remember visiting a friend whose father had been chronically depressed for about fifteen years. He lived with his wife, but was scarcely present in the relationship. Often he sat in a slumped position and simply stared into the distance. On this occasion we had all gone to the beach together and there he was sitting slumped forward in his usual way. My friend and I decided to take a walk on the beach, and we invited him along. As we began our walk he remained bent over and wasn't involved in the conversation. But as we moved down the beach away from his wife, he slowly began to listen a little to what we were talking about; eventually he made a contribution. We moved on, and he began to walk in the water a little instead of on the sand. Slowly we approached a nude beach, and as we do so our conversation picked up and we're laughing. Slowly his posture changed and he began to smile and then to laugh. By the time we reach this nude beach he was a full and forthright human being. He was part of the conversation, part of the day, part of the physicality of the environment; he was wonderful. But as we later walked back down the beach his posture began to change again—from the upright to the slumped. He became increasingly quiet, and when he finally sat down—or shall I say, fell in a heap by his wife—he was that fully depressed individual again. Let me just complete this by saying that I think therapeutically, if we could only keep him at the other end of the beach, he would be fine. But how do we change that relationship with his wife, for obviously this is importantly a problem of the relationship between them. Can our walks give him the resources that would alter her moves in the dance, and thus his in the future?

M. Elkaïm: Firstly, you said very clearly, it's not just the wife. The wife is part of a larger context, and what you saw was that when he was close to her, he seemed depressed, when he was far away, he seemed less depressed. Perhaps she's not the one who makes him look depressed, rather she's part of the context in which he functions as depressed. So you see, the way we will function will be like this: we will ask ourselves, "What is the dance they dance together?" Generally that dance isn't only the revolving door that each one of them pushes, it is also the context with their parents, her parents, his parents, their children, work, and in the situation you describe, the friends, the water, the nude part of the beach, the whole context. So for me, these will be the assemblages I have to take into account, and I will see how I can use myself in that context to try to change the way they relate. And I'm going to be multiple also, I'm going to be allied with her and with him at the same time, and I will do this honestly and completely. I am in it, honestly, authentically, and people feel that. My aim obviously is to make them better, but I'm not going to think, "Aha, I'm going to do this so that will happen." I don't think like that. I think, "Aha, he feels that way and I am touched that he feels that way. How can I use myself in that context so that he can feel at the same time understood, but with an alternative that he doesn't see now?" In that couple, there are a lot of possibilities. One is to ask myself, for example, why does she need a depressed man? Perhaps she's a lady who was mostly welcomed when she was taking care of others. Perhaps she's a lady who didn't blossom enough and who is stopped at part of her growth where she needs to take care of others. Then perhaps I can work with them and help her to be more multiple, to accept that in her there is also a child who wants to be cared for and an adult who wants to do things on her own. You often hear about women whose husbands die when they are in their seventies, and the women are in their sixties, and suddenly they begin to live completely different lives because they weren't aware of certain aspects of themselves. They didn't know how to sign a check, they didn't know how to do a lot of things, and then they begin to create a lot of new things because they have an opportunity to grow. Then for example, I would ask myself, "What is happening in this man's context which is amplifying something in him which is perhaps genetic or perhaps organic, but which isn't condemning, because when he is on the other side of the beach, he's fine." So I will work with what I call the function of his behavior in that context, and look at how I can change the relationship in that context so that the function won't be useful any longer. If it becomes useless, then the symptom will perhaps change. For me, the idea of function remains important: even if I don't think in terms of a function of a symptom in a real system, I think in terms of a function of a symptom in an interrelationship of constructs, an interrelationship of assemblages.

K. Gergen: So often in therapy, you only have a part of the system; you only have the single individual, and not the wife there with whom you can work on the issues. Then the question is, how is it that you can enable that individual, that single individual, that depressed person to go back to that wife's context in such a way that her patterns are going to be altered? It's at that point, I think, that it may not be sufficient that you can generate the alternative moves in the dance of therapy that will recreate him. He must have the resources for recreating also his wife, and the question is whether at that point, some of the sort of theoretics which we share couldn't also be useful as a way of trying to give that person a sense of what's possible, that he also is helping to create his own depression. He's part of a system which indeed is self-creating.

M. Elkaïm: I would say that it all depends on the philosophy of the therapist. If he's a therapist who thinks that he can make his patients, his clients, therapists themselves, then he will teach them, he will explain to them. However, he'll also be aware that it's not in the explanation that the change will happen, but also in the relationship with him, perhaps because the patient or client will act towards him as if he were the wife, and the therapist acting differently than the wife acts will open up new paths to that man. So I think it is possible to act in a way where we offer not only theoretical knowledge to the client, but also a different kind of affective feeling.

K. Gergen: I very much agree. My suggestion here is only part of the more general concern I have for expanding the range of what we take to be legitimate therapeutic actions. I don't wish to give up anything so much as to expand our definition of what we take to be therapy, and specifically to do so by thinking about it from a constructionist standpoint.

9

Postmodernism, The Relational Self, And Beyond

Michael Hoyt interviews Kenneth Gergen

Michael Hoyt is a major contributor to the theory and practice of brief therapy. He is a senior staff psychologist at the Kaiser Permanente Medical Center in San Rafael, CA, and a faculty member at the University of California School of Medicine in San Francisco. Hoyt is the author of numerous books and articles, including Some Stories are Better than Others (2000), and Interviews with Brief Therapy Experts (2001). He is also the editor of Constructive Therapies, Vols. 1 & 2 (1994, 1996), and the Handbook of Constructive Therapies (1998).

M. Hoyt: How do you conceptualize the "self," and how does this change as we move from a modern to a postmodern perspective?

K. Gergen: For purposes of contrast, let's start with the tradition we inherit in the West, one which posits some form of inner essence. Whether we are speaking of Christian religion and its belief in a soul; Romanticists of the past century, with their championing of passion, inspiration, or *elan vital*; recent existentialist thinkers and their emphasis on conscious choice; or the belief of modernists in reason or cognition—all begin with the assumption of an essential core of the self. It is this essence that constitutes one's being and without which one would be something less than human.

Speaking as a social constructionist, we may view all these perspectives as culturally and historically situated. It is not that they are mistaken, somehow failing to see the self as it truly is. The mistake is perhaps in presuming that we can determine "what truly is." The words we use to describe our being are not simply pictures of what exists, not maps of a territory. Rather, they construct us as this or that, and in doing so serve as logics for action. I think it is this de-essentializing that is the major ingredient of the move from the modern to postmodern conception of self. At the same time, there are efforts—including my own—to reconceptualize the self in a more relational way. That is, rather than defining the person in terms of an essence that stands independent of others, the effort is to understand us as thoroughly entwined.

M. Hoyt: If the self is socially constructed, is there something essential that may be shaped or influenced, but is not created *sui generis* ? I'm thinking, for example, of Stern's studies of infant development and Margaret Mahler's (Bergman & Pine, 1975) ideas about the "psycho logical birth of the infant." Other writers, such as Singer and Salovey have suggested that one's sense of self is remembered, organized or influenced by cognitive-affective processes.

K. Gergen: Again, the challenge for the constructionist is to avoid pronouncements about what is essential. This is not to say that the constructionist doesn't participate in culture, and would not use words like soul, intentional choice, cognition, and the like. Rather, it is to recognize that when we use these utterances we are participating in a particular set of cultural traditions, and not pronouncing truth beyond culture and history. To say "I love you" is not then a description of a mental state; it is active participation in a deeply valued form of relationship.

To deal with your question more directly, I don't want to say either that *there is* or *is not* something essential in the head to be shaped or influenced. We could debate this till the end of time. Rather, let's ask what hangs on the question for different social or cultural practices. What will follow if I take one route in a conversation as opposed to another? As I mentioned previously, we have a substantial tradition of essentialism, giving an affirmative answer to your question. So for me as a scholar, I scarcely succeed in pressing our cultural potentials forward if I simply say, yet once again, "We are emotional beings," or "cognitive beings" or "intentional beings."

As I suggested, one of my central interests has been to generate a new sense of what it is to be a person, a sense of what I call a "relational self." The hope is to transform the meaning of what it is to be a self—to have an identity, emotion, memory, and the like—so that we can understand it as constituted within relationship. Vygotsky and Bakhtin are useful as first steps in this direction, as are Mead and Bruner. However, in each of these cases there remains a strong commitment to an individual subjectivity that precedes relatedness. My hope is to go beyond this work by positing relatedness as the essential matrix, out of which a conception of self (or identity, emotion, etc.) is born, objectified, and embedded within action.

From a relational perspective, we might say, for example, that the term "emotion" is a constructed category. However, we use these terms, such as "I am angry" "I am happy," to carry out the rituals that constitute cultural life. We perform the emotions and these performances are never cut away from a relational dance or scenario. We participate in the dance together, and without the dance there would be no occasion for the performance. In this sense, it is *we* who possess the emotion. Much of this is spelled out in my book, Realities and Relationships.

M. Hoyt: This is very consistent with the interactionist notion that the basic unit of analysis is at least two people, as I recently heard Jay Haley express it, as well as the idea that "the mind is not in the head" (Maturana

& Varela, 1987). In your view, where is the unconscious? Is the term useful? Is there a self outside (beyond, below) narrative?

K. Gergen: It follows from what I just said that whether we posit an unconscious mind is optional. There is nothing about whatever we are that makes this kind of description necessary. Our beliefs in the unconscious as a reality are also culturally and historically situated, growing most recently from the soil of 19th-century Romanticism. However, whether the term is useful or not is a very interesting one. It is not useful if what we mean by the term is that the concept gives us an accurate description or "real insight" into human functioning. However, if what we mean by "useful" is viewed in terms of social functioning, where does it get us in our relations to speak of the unconscious? In this case I think the answer would be very multifaceted.

M. Hoyt: How so?

K. Gergen: For example, the concept has been very useful in augmenting our tendency to place moral judgment on the deviant in society. Rather than simply placing moral blame on the rapist, child molester, or murderer—typically leading to punishment, the concept of the unconscious adds to our cultural repertoire by enabling us to see the deviant as in some sense "ill." We think increasingly, then, about ways to restore the individual to full functioning (as opposed to forms of punishment that will virtually ensure their remaining deviant). There is much more that could be said on behalf of the concept of the unconscious.

However, there are also problems inherent in the way we use the term, and I guess I find these more compelling than the positive account. Here I am speaking of the many critiques of the assumption of the unconscious, for example, when it is used to reduce all problems to the intrapsychic level of the individual, to obliterate consideration of cultural and economic conditions, to champion the authority of the all-knowing doctor (in contrast to the ignorant patient), to reinforce the medical model of illness, and to provide the individual excuses for all forms of brutishness.

M. Hoyt: How do you define therapy? Is that the right word? What might be an alternative?

K. Gergen: I would prefer not to define it. Rather, let's say that we find ourselves at this time in cultural history engaged in a range of interrelated conversations in which the concept of therapy plays a very significant role. The precise meaning of the term is contested, and it should ideally remain so. To legislate in this case would be to stop the conversation, oppress the many voices, and arbitrarily and misleadingly freeze history.

M. Hoyt: How do you currently see the therapeutic endeavor?

K. Gergen: My preference in this conversation is to view therapy as a process of constructing meaning. To be sure, we exist in what we commonly call "real-world conditions"—biological, material, economic, and the like. However, in the main what we take to be the successes and failures in our lives, the worthwhile and the worthless, the satisfying and the frustrating, are byproducts of human meaning. It is not so much "how things are" that is important but how we interpret them that will typically bring us into therapy.

For example, a physical touch may itself be unremarkable; however, in different frames of meaning it may spark a sense of friendly support, move one to ecstasy, or incite litigation for harassment. A blow to the chin will send a family member in search of a therapist, but will move a boxer to change his tactics. With this emphasis in place, we are invited to see effective therapy as a transformation in meaning. However, as you can see from the preceding remarks, I don't see this transformation principally as a cognitive event. Rather, it is an alteration in action, relying importantly on language but not at all limited to language.

M. Hoyt: As therapy moves more into postmodern context, what are the continuities from past tradition and practice, and what new directions should we consider? It would be perhaps premature and too specific to propose a curriculum, but what do you see as the major issues and challenges?

K. Gergen: These are very complicated issues and we could talk at length. For now, however, let me focus on just one aspect of what many see as the postmodern condition, and its particular implications for therapeutic practice. As I tried to describe in The Saturated Self, the communication technologies of this century bring us into confrontation with a vastly expanded range of others—both in terms of physical presence and vicarious figures of the media. Our otherwise parochial worlds become shattered by the intrusion of a multiplicity of opinions, values, attitudes, personalities, visions, and ways of life. At the same time, there has been an increasing tendency for various groups to generate common consciousness. Again, the technologies allow otherwise voiceless people to organize, develop common goals, consider entitlements, and so on. Under these conditions of increasing pluralism, it is very difficult for any therapeutic school to claim overall or ubiquitous authority. To reduce all problems, for example, to early family conditions, conditioned responses, or deficits in self-regard not only seems excessively parochial, but in a certain sense tyrannical.

M. Hoyt: The death of an orthodoxy makes it difficult to organize a counter-orthodoxy.

K. Gergen: How then does therapeutic practice respond to these conditions? Of course, the most common practice among therapists is simply to "go eclectic." Rather than continuing in the often narrow practices favored in their training, they continue to explore, learn, adapt, and eventually develop multi-layered approaches. In my view, a constructionist orientation favors just this kind of practice, but as well furnishes such practice with a needed sense of integration and purpose.

M. Hoyt: I prefer the term multi-layered or multi-theoretical rather than eclectic. Being multiply informed is important, but to me eclectic sometimes seems like a cross between electric and chaotic, a directionless hodgepodge of techniques.

K. Gergen: Good point. We could also use the term polyvocal, which better fits the metaphor of conversation. In any case, the greater the range of vocabularies available to the therapist, the greater his or her efficacy within wide-ranging client relationships. At the same time, the constructionist therapist is drawn to the use-value of these various vocabularies (words and actions) as they are developed in the therapeutic relationship, and extended to further relationships outside. How well do the vocabularies travel, and what do they do to and for people's lives as they are pressed into action?

M. Hoyt: Holy hermeneutics! If modernism gave us "ontological insecurity," postmodernism could produce a panic attack! As Sheila McNamee and you (1992, p. 2) have commented, "Little confidence now remains in the optimistic program of scientifically grounded progress toward identifying 'problems' and providing 'cures.'" With conventional standards of what is right no longer valid compasses, what suggestions do you have for therapists as we search for (and co-create) therapeutic realities with our clients? Any guides for the perplexed?

K. Gergen: At the outset, I think we must all remain humble and interdependent in the face of the plural worlds of the real and the good. This is not the time to look to a new guru who can remove our perplexities; we must together work toward new visions. With this said, my own preference is for a therapeutic approach that appreciates the force of local realities, but within an expanded context of connection. By this, I mean that the therapist would not begin with a single set of criteria as to what constitutes an effective intervention or a cure. Rather, he or she would be maximally sensitive to how such matters are defined within the local communities. What are the standards for judging satisfaction or dissatisfaction within the most immediate relationships at hand? At the same time, the therapist must remain concerned with the fuller range of relationships in which the immediate case is embedded. Meaning within the local condition is ultimately dependent upon broader cultural context. Again, this won't lead to a single standard. But the point is to allow the mix of standards into the therapeutic conversation.

M. Hoyt: This gets at one of the challenges of a multicultural society, where different groups have different mores and standards. How do we steer between the Scylla of a Balkanized, "anything goes" separatism and the Charybdis of a colonization by the dominant culture?

K. Gergen: It is in the mix of voices, it seems to me, that we find the answer—in the blending, appropriation, and paradox that result when we talk meaningfully together. This does not mean that anything goes; not at all. For example, a therapist could confront a family in which a certain degree of incestual activity or physical abuse was quite fully tolerated—not really a problem as they see it.

In my view, it wouldn't be the therapist's immediate task to deconstruct the family's system of values or beliefs (legal issues notwithstanding). However, given the ultimate interdependence of this family on the broader array of cultural meanings, therapy might usefully be directed to coordinating the local family meanings (and actions) with those of the dominant society. In effect, their private activities as a family would ideally be modified by their interchange with the views of the dominant culture. In many cases of incest, for example, the child does not suffer until she (or he) realizes the cultural stigma attached to such activity. This confrontation can generate a lifetime of anguish. In effect, it is the therapist's task in this case to create a meaningful interchange between the local meanings and those of the surrounding culture.

M. Hoyt: In the last chapter of Therapy as Social Construction (McNamee & Gergen, 1992), Efran and Clarfield review what they consider to be "sense and nonsense" in constructionist therapy. They evoke Coyn's (1982) term "epistobabble" and note, to use their words (p. 200), that some critics dismiss such therapies as "little more than recombinations of familiar reframing and team observation techniques already in use." They question whether constructionist lingo will prove any more substantive or long-lived than a dozen earlier infatuations. What do you see as truly different and likely to endure?

K. Gergen: It's difficult to understand why Efran and Clarfield were so hostile to almost everyone unfortunate enough to draw their gaze. I think disagreements can be useful and wonderful means toward new visions, but it seems primitive to me to abuse your colleagues in the ways they selected.

M. Hoyt: Beyond the mean-spiritedness of their critique, what is added?

K. Gergen: In my view, the importance of social constructionism to current therapeutic theory and practice is that it enables many practitioners to 1) articulate emerging beliefs and practices in such a way that they can more clearly see their advantages over what was taught within the modernist tradition; 2) appreciate the similarities between their practices and what many others are doing in the field; and 3) understand how their orientation is related to a vast range of cultural changes, including major intellectual transformations in the academy and changes in societal life patterns.

I don't see constructionism as offering just another model of therapy, "silver bullet" cure, a specialized vocabulary, or a new set of "musts." Rather, I see constructionism as inherent in a vast array of conversations taking place around the world—conversations that bring people together over pressing issues of common concern. To be sure, constructionist discussions cannot do everything one might wish. However, they do raise fundamental questions about long-cherished traditions in Western culture. Given the rapid changes taking place in meanings, values, and practices, and the enormous conflicts among meaning systems around the world, constructionist ideas are likely to remain relevant for some time.

M. Hoyt: Raising consciousness via the question, as Watzlawick put it, "How real is real, (1994a, 1996, 1993) and that reality is "invented" (1984), could have, if not a humbling effect, at least suggest some pause and respect. It could open dialogic space, one would hope. In this regard, let me note that in your Foreword (1993) to Friedman's <u>The New Language of Change</u>, you comment that this shift constructionist shift entails a "formidable change of sense, in which there is the suspicion of all reality posits...coupled with a related distrust of the authoritative voice."(x) Given that we cannot stand outside the equation, how can we practice therapy without imposing our values or ethics?

K. Gergen: There is no therapy that stands outside values or ethics; even the most politically neutral therapist is acting for good or ill by some standard. Given this fact, many therapists are drawn to the conclusion that therapy should thereby operate as advocacy. If we are bound to be advocates in any case, it is reasoned, then why not be clear and open about what it is we stand for and what we are against, and use therapy to build a better society?

In certain ways I am drawn to this kind of thinking; it is surely an improvement over the old modernist attempt to step outside the conversation by declaring value neutrality. However, I also worry about the implications of the advocacy orientation if it is fully extended. Can you imagine the results for the profession if we split into hundreds of political encampments the gay, the gray, the lesbian, the black, the Chicano, the Asian, and so on—each with suspicion or antipathy toward the other? This would be multi-culturalism gone mad. If we separate along moral-political lines, not only do we diminish the possibility for dialogue and communality but we also generate a therapeutic world of all against all.

Perhaps you can see again why I favor forms of therapy that enable people to speak in many voices, to comprehend the paradoxes in their own values, to appreciate the positive force of many local intelligibilities. The challenge here would not be to locate the one right position, ethic, or political ideal; nor would it be to suppress informed political action. Rather, it is to enable people to move with greater fluidity in the world, with a greater potential perhaps for coordinating the otherwise alienated as opposed to eradicating the opposition.

M. Hoyt: You have written eloquently (1994) about ways that the therapeutic professions have developed and disseminated a language of mental deficit—a language that creates hierarchies, dependencies, and endless ways of constructing the self as deficient. We now seem to have a flood of new self disorders, such as multiple personality disorder, narcissistic disorder, borderline disorder, codependency, and the like. How can we redress this situation? Can we reeducate the profession, the media, and the public?

K. Gergen: I do think the therapeutic community has provided an invaluable resource to people over the years, and particularly as traditional social bonds have eroded. As families, committed friendships, and communities disappear into the past, therapists continue to "be there" for support, insight, renewal, and the like. And given our technologies of saturation, this trend is only likely to continue.

However, if there is one marked failure of the therapeutic communities, it is not in terms of outcome evaluation. (Personally, I think outcome evaluations are no more than window dressing for a given school of therapy, and the entire concept is misleading.) Rather, there has been a profound disservice in generating an enormous set of concepts through which people can see themselves as deficient. Worse, these vocabularies are self-serving; when people come to believe they possess these "diseases" or "failings" a therapist is required for "cure."

To be sure, education can be an important means to the re-empowering of the public. However, this first means a major change within the therapeutic community. That is, it is first necessary to get our own house in order. Family therapists have been in the vanguard of criticism of diagnosis; however, there is simultaneously a move within the family arena to develop an entirely new range of deficit categories, namely, relational diagnostics. And there are still the clinical psychology and psychiatric professions for whom these deficit categories are no less than maps of the real world.

Coupled with this self-critical effort, and perhaps more realistic, is the decoupling of diagnosis and third-party billing procedures. So long as diagnostic categories are necessary for insurance payments, the professions will capitulate. This procedure can and should be reversed. After all, we have learned to live with "no-fault" divorce processes. Why can the same logic not apply in the case of difficulties in living? The day is also soon coming when activist ex-mental patients will bring lawsuits against therapists for such unjustifiable and injurious classification. Perhaps such litigation can speed the process of change.

M. Hoyt: Some cultures, such as the traditional Balinese (Suryani and Jensen, 1993), create or construct "selves" that in some ways resemble the condition we call "multiple personality disorder." Other writers, such as Glass (1993) in Shattered Selves: Multiple Personality in a Postmodern World, are very critical of postmodern conceptions of the self, arguing that true MPD is a fragmentation of self resulting from horrible childhood abuse and that such individuals suffer greatly for having to live without a firm identity. How do you see the relationship between a postmodern view of self and multiple personality disorder?

K. Gergen: First, the assumptions embraced by Glass, that there simply are "MPD" persons in the world, and that they chiefly suffer from the lack of a firm identity, are exactly the kind of assumptions that I see as detrimental to the culture. Such presumptions not only serve to objectify the illness, and to suggest that others may also possess this particular infirmity, but as well imply that there is something privileged in a state of unified and coherent being. In a certain sense, then, this kind of analysis is part of the problem.

Now this is not to doubt that Glass confronts clients who are in deep pain, and that they can understand themselves in just the way he describes. But there are many other ways in which one's personality can be rendered meaningful, many alternative conceptions that can be generated to what he is authoritatively classified as MPD. And many of these alternatives would, in my view, be far more promising for the client (and society), as they move from therapeutic relations into daily life. For example, why not explore the advantages of multiple personalities, or the possibility that some people are maximally attuned to the many voices and potentials we carry with us?

There is also a certain genre of postmodern writing that provides just such a promise. If one feels split among selves, torn between competing tendencies, capable of multiple personalities, this literature suggests that such a condition may be the newly emerging cultural form. And it is not to be lamented, but explored for its potential riches. Contributions to this genre would include the work of Jim Wertsch (1991) in psychology, and Peggy Penn (1985; Penn & Frankfurt, 1994) in family therapy, and Carl Tomm (1992) in family therapy.

M. Hoyt: Reading through some of the chapters in The Saturated Self in the rapid way you recommend (1991, p. 49) did produce the existentially dizzying, almost disorienting "multiphrenic" effect that, the complexity of (post)modern life exceeds our cognitive grasp. In multiphrenia, what will provide a sense of stability/identity/self?

K. Gergen: As you might guess from what I just said, we might ask, what is necessarily wrong with instability and fragmentation? These are, after all, negative labels for conditions that might also be described as fascinating, exciting, and transformative, on the one hand, or multifaceted or richly complex on the other. The opposite of instability could be viewed as a boring and oppressive status quo, while the opposite of fragmentation might be seen as rigidity and narrow-mindedness. This is not to say that I wish to abandon the quest for stability and simplicity. There are days and hours in which I long for it. But I can also understand these wishes in terms of my immersion in a cultural history in which these conditions are valued, and understand that these yearnings are not something fundamental, deeply ingrained in nature. (I read recently of a musician who felt more at home "on the road" than he did living in a stationary dwelling.) Thus, while we may yearn, we must also be aware that we are not bound by our history. That idea in itself I find helpful.

M. Hoyt: What will character mean in a postmodern world? How do we understand ethics and integrity (acting consistent with one's values) if we are "saturated" and "polymorphous"?

K. Gergen: I do feel that postmodern writers have been unfairly criticized for their inability to support firm moral values, for their "relativism," as it is often put. For who in this century, outside the highly parochial and fanatic, are willing to declare what is good and right for all people for all time? The postmodern writers are too frequently scapegoated for the incapacities of those who criticize. The critics want foundational values, but cannot locate the foundations; then they attack the postmodernist for not providing them.

I also feel that in their explorations of multiple selves and constructed realities, postmodern writings open important new vistas in our comprehension of morality and for practices more fully suited to living together in a world of differences. They suggest, for one, that we should cease looking to a slate of ideals, ethical foundations, a code of justice, or canons or morality in order to create "good persons" or a "just society." High-sounding words and phrases themselves require nothing in the way of subsequent action, and may be interpreted in so many ways that even the most violent oppression can be justified on the basis of the most glowing ideals. I believe we should turn away from abstract justifications and look to ourselves in the process of relationship. For it is out of these relationships that we generate the hells for ourselves that we term injustice, oppression, immorality, and so on.

M. Hoyt: I take what you're saying suggests a higher moral challenge. If we give up the notion of an "ultimate truth," then we have to take full responsibility for all of our constructions and actions, and realize that others are just as entitled to theirs.

K. Gergen: Your comment takes us part of the way, but there is more: Faced now with ourselves in relationship, we may then together ask about the kinds of practices that bring about these alienated conditions, and the ways in which these practices might be altered. It is not a matter of each individual taking responsibility for his or her actions, but of people in relationship inquiring into their patterns of interchange, and the kinds of worlds they would like to create together.

This kind of thinking also inspired my work with Sheila McNamee (McNamee and Gergen, 1992) on what we call " relational responsibility." Here we are raising criticisms with the traditional view of holding individuals morally responsible for problematic actions, and trying to develop some conversational resources that might enable people to explore the forms of relatedness in which the problematic action takes place. The major challenge we face is in sustaining the kinds of relationships out of which meaning can continuously be made. We must be responsible to relatedness itself, for without forms of generative relationship the very capacity to envision "the good" "the valuable," and the "worthy" begin to erode.

M. Hoyt: I expect that this may be related to the experience you wrote about (1994b, 76-77) in "The Limits of Pure Critique." Let me quote at length:

> At the beginning of a three-day conference, the organizers arranged a confrontation pitting radical constructivism (as represented by Ernst von Glazerfeld) against social constructionism (which I was to profess). The subsequent critiques were unsparing, the defenses unyielding, and as the audience was drawn into the debate polarization rapidly took place. Voices became agitated, critique turned ad hominem, anger and alienation mounted. As the moderator called a halt to the proceedings, I began to see the three days before me as an eternity...Here, Tomm asked if von Glazerfeld and I would be willing to be publicly interviewed. Most important, would we be willing to do so as the other? Uneasily, we agreed....Our exposure to each other did allow each of us to absorb aspects of the other intellectual views, attitudes, values which we now carried with us as potentials. The initial question was whether we were willing and able to give these potentials credible voice. Through an extended series of questions, carefully and sensitively addressed, Tomm was able to elicit "the other within." Playing the other's identity,

we discussed issues of theory, views of the other, self-doubts, fears, personal relationships, feelings about the conference and so on.

The results of the procedure were striking. As both we and the audience learned, we could communicate intelligibly and sympathetically from within the other's framework. Each could give voice to the rationality of the other. Further, the binary was successfully broken. Rather than a showdown between competing epistemologies, the debate could be understood within the context of a long interpersonal history, imbricated friendships, private aspirations and doubts, the demands of public debate and so on. A new level of discussion ensued. The conference was thereafter marked by its civility of interchange; there was expression without domination, careful listening and sensitive reply. No, this did not mean a resolution of differences; the lines of difference remained clear. However, it did allow the exploration to move forward, and with the resulting emergency of new complexities, the old yearnings for victory and defeat. heroes and villains, receded from view.

When I recently asked David Epston what he would like to ask you, he called my attention to this passage and said he would ask, "Where do you think you will take such developments both in the realm of ideas and everyday life from here?" Pray tell?

K. Gergen: On the theoretical side, you might imagine from my earlier comments that my major concern is with expanding conceptions of relatedness. I call this "relational theory," a project that begins with <u>Realities and Relationships</u> (Gergen, 1994), but has since expanded in several directions. Given the quotation you just cited, you can imagine that such theorizing is also directed toward more practical domains—including therapy, education, organizational management, and politics. The challenge is to bring about metaphors, stories, distinctions, images, and so on that don't so much reflect what is, but create what can be.

I also work with various therapists, organizational consultants, global businesses, and the like to develop practices that embody a relational perspective. With some friends, we created The Taos Institute (www.taosinstitute.net), an institute centered in New Mexico that brings theorists and practitioners together to work on cutting-edge issues in relational process. Perhaps the most wonderful thing about this kind of work is that you never feel you are alone—fully responsible for all the ideas, plans, practices, outcomes, and so on. The work becomes lighter, more joyous, and more optimistic. Also, I find the creative potential of dialogue is just enormous, and the challenge of developing new forms of dialogue very exciting.

M. Hoyt: The work of Michel Foucault (1975, 1978, 1980), especially his views on the relationship of power and knowledge, has influenced many therapists working within narrative constructive frameworks. Not everyone is so impressed, however. Camille Paglia (p. 174) has written: "Foucault's biggest fans are not among the majority of philosophers, historians, and sociologists, who usually perceive his glaring inadequacies of knowledge and argument, but among well-meaning but foggy humanists, who virtually never have the intellectual and scholarly preparation to critique Foucault competently. The more you know, the less you are impressed by Foucault." What do you think of Foucault's contribution, and what do you think of Paglia's dismissal?

K. Gergen: To pick up on an earlier theme, I don't look to Foucault or any other writer now for "the truth," nor for a perfect and well-defended logic, new set of foundations, ideals, or premises for a new life. Rather, from my constructionist background, I am inclined to ask whether a given piece of writing can offer resources for the kinds of conversations in which I now find myself. If I borrow from the words, the metaphors, the logics within the writing, what happens now to my various relationships?

In this sense I have found certain of Foucault's concepts very useful—as have many others, and scarcely "foggy humanists." Foucault's writings help us do things in conversations that we could less easily or not possibly do before. No, I don't find all of Foucault so useful; by contemporary American standards the writing is sometimes opaque, incoherent, and mystifying, and his major analyses of history quite selective. However, in his critiques of traditional conceptions of power, in his emphasis on the relationship of language to power, and his discussion of the delimiting effects of various professional discourses on society, he has been enormously useful.

M. Hoyt: How about Paglia?

K. Gergen: Along these same lines, I don't find Paglia so very helpful. If I put her discourse into action, I am more likely to find myself in a set of conflictual and aggressive relationships. To borrow her discourse often leads to a form of relationship in which mutual annihilation is the implicit end. Do we need more of this in our world?

M. Hoyt: In "The Social Construction of Narrative Accounts," you and Mary Gergen (M. Gergen & Gergen, 1984; see also K. J. Gergen & Gergen, 1986, 1988; M. M. Gergen & Gergen, 1993) discuss progressive, stabilizing, and regressive narratives. You also comment (p. 177) that what might look "regressive" (or a downward spiraling) could be part of a forward movement in life, or a larger homeostasis. As the French say, to make an omelet you have first to break the eggs. With multiphrenia and such a complexity of competing goals, how is primacy established? What dialectic, what values guide complex, competing choices?

K. Gergen: Perhaps I can answer this in a way that will clarify what I was trying to say regarding value positions. It seems to me that in the Western tradition we are supposed to possess some personal logic, set of values, or well-considered aim in life that should guide us through such complex situations. Yet, it is just such a view that social constructionism calls into question. For a constructionist, logic values, aims, and the like are more effectively viewed as positions in a conversation. The languages of logic, values, and so on do not cause action; they are action in themselves. And if they occur privately (what we have traditionally considered "in the mind"), nothing necessarily follows in terms of "choices" (another term heavily weighted by our psychologistic and individualistic tradition).

Further, as I have tried to stress, we might usefully see intelligible action in terms of its place within patterns of relationship. In this context, rather than trying to work out a fully developed set of priorities abstracted from concrete conditions of relationship, it seems more promising from a constructionist standpoint to immerse oneself more fully in one's expanded array of relationships. I like as an illustration the actions of the unmarried pregnant adolescents interviewed in Gilligan's (1982) landmark work, In a Different Voice. When confronted with the difficult question of abortion, they didn't resort to abstract principles, but sought out relationships. They engaged in multiple conversations -with friends, parents, clergy, the potential father, and so on. From the engagement in relationship, decisions emerged from the matrix of relevant voices.

M. Hoyt: There seem to be two opposite trends occurring simultaneously. One involves the emergence of the "relational self," and the other a tendency toward greater isolation and loneliness. Do you agree? How do you understand the "relational self" and what is happening more generally in our society?

K. Gergen: There are a number of ways to go with this question; let me try only one. On a theoretical level I want to propose that all selves are relational, and always have been. Unless a feral child or severely brain damaged, even the physically isolated individual (for example, the elderly shut-in or the prisoner in solitary confinement) is immersed in relationship. Without a history of relationship there would indeed be no way of making sense of one's condition.

At the same time, I think you are absolutely correct in your observation that people are more physically isolated than ever before. This is part of the irony of The Saturated Self. The very technologies that bring the teeming array of images, voices, dramas, logics, and so on into our lives (e.g., television, radio, mass print, telephone, VCRs, personal computers), are also the same technologies that allow us to exist quite pleasantly without others' physical presence. So we are more multiply related but more physically alone. I worry a great deal about this trend; the consequences for society are profound. A major interest for me now is whether we might use some of these same technologies (and especially computer networks) to generate new forms of community.

M. Hoyt: The information and networking possibilities are thrilling, but I hope virtual reality and cybersex won't replace older forms! In We've Had a Hundred Years of Psychotherapy and the World is Getting Worse, James Hillman and Michael Ventura argue that the pendulum has swung too far toward the individual self, producing a narcissistic preoccupation, and call for a greater identification with society. Some religious and spiritual practices also advocate connection to humanity or nature as part of a larger sense of self. How does this fit with your idea of the relational self?

K. Gergen: I entirely agree with the thesis that the pendulum has swung too far toward the individual self. A narcissistic preoccupation is only one of the problematic consequences. I'm less positive about a solution which requires a greater identification with society, as it suggests that I exist separate from society. "Here I am," and over there is "the society" to which I should related. But if I am also part of society, where do I end and does society begin?

At the same time, I resonate with some spiritual, religious, and ecological movements which generate a sense of our greater relatedness. A great deal of my recent work explores the ways in which we are always already constituted within relationship. As I mentioned earlier, I try to focus on various ways in which to be a self, to have an idea, to possess an emotion is to be acting out of and into relatedness. I am also working with therapists and organizational consultants to bring these kinds of ideas into practice, and with an artist and a film maker in trying to give this consciousness a visual dimension.

M. Hoyt: I want to ask you about your remarks at the end of your keynote speech at the Therapeutic Conversations 2 conference in Washington, D.C when you commented that "We don't live in narratives, we live with them," and spoke of moving "beyond stories to relatedness itself." It's hard to talk about what is beyond words. At the risk of asking an oxymoronic question, would you expound on the ineffable lightness of being?

K. Gergen: My major aim in that conclusion was to rise above the excessive focus on language as an end in itself. Too often it is presumed that if an individual learns to "re-narrate," he or she has essentially undergone a "change of mind." We try as therapists to generate new meanings, new narratives, new constructions, as if a new set of words will "do the trick," because the individual now thinks differently. In fact, I tend to talk that way myself at times. However, this is to miss the ultimate concern, which is relatedness itself—out of which meanings are generated. In effect, relations precede meaning.

Yet, it is at this point that we begin to approach a mystery—a movement toward what we might see as a spiritual consciousness. To begin with, as I try to speak about moving beyond stories to relatedness itself I find myself resisting clarity, wanting rather to move by metaphor and intimation. This is because in the struggle to be clear about relational process—from which all that is meaningful emerges—I realize my capacity to speak such process is limited by the language available to me. I cannot exit "the house of language" to understand it from the outside.

Further, when I think of "getting it right" about the nature of relational process, I realize that to draw any final conclusions is to terminate the flow of conversation. If we "pin it down," we also close down the very process of dialogue that we so value. So, rather than trying to get clear on the nature of relationship, I look to metaphors, ambiguous concepts, or parables.

The plot thickens: Some years ago I played with the concept of a *relational sublime*. Here I borrowed heavily from the Romanticist idea of a mental condition which transcends the capacity of rational comprehension. The Romanticists often used the term to depict a condition in which one sensed the incomprehensible scope and power of nature—a towering waterfall, a snow capped alpine mountain, a roaring ocean. 1 rather liked these images, and felt that they might help us to develop an awesome sense of ourselves as fully immersed in relatedness—all humanity, all that is given in nature. Yet, as we begin to consider these possibilities, we also begin to realize that the very processes from which all that is meaningful and significant emerges is ultimately beyond our comprehension, beyond words. Is this not a theme also located in many religious traditions—which the vast creative power giving rise to all that exists is beyond human comprehension?

Might we enter a promising and profound space of understanding if we viewed the creation and sustenance of relationship as sacred? These ideas are developed a little further in a book edited by Chris Hermans and his colleagues, Social Construction and Theology.

M. Hoyt: We're all in this together. Thank you.

References

Al-Issa, I. (Ed.) (1995). Handbook of Culture and Mental Illness: An International Perspective. Washington, D.C.: International Universities Press.

American Psychiatric Association (1994) Diagnostic and Statistical Manual of Mental Disorders (4th ed.). Washington, D.C.

Andersen, T. (1991) The Reflecting Team: Dialogues and Dialogues about the Dialogues. New York: Norton.

_____ (1995) Reflecting processes; acts of informing and forming; you can borrow my eyes but you must not take them away from me! In S. Friedman (Ed.) The Reflecting Team in Action. New York: Guilford Press, p. 11-38.

Andersen, T. (1997) Gaining more therapist sensitivity through a common research process of client and therapist. Zeitschrift für systemische Therapie, 15, (3), p. 160-167.

Anderson, H. (1997) Conversation, Language and Possibilities. A Postmodern Approach to Psychotherapy. New York: Basic Books.

Anderson, H. & Goolishian H.A. (1992) The client is the expert: a not-knowing approach to therapy. In S. McNamee, K.J. Gergen, (Eds.) Therapy as Social Construction. Thousand Oaks, CA: Sage, p. 25-38.

Anderson, H. & Goolishian, H.A. (1992a) Telling stories and not-knowing in Therapies. In Systeme, 6, p. 15-21.

Anderson, H. & Goolishian, H.A. (1992b) The client is the expert: a not-knowing approach to therapy. In Zeitschrift für systemische Therapie, 10, (3), p. 176-189.

Aponte, H.J. (1995) Bread and Spirit: Therapy with the New Poor. New York: Norton.

Ashback, C. & Schermer, V.L., (1987) Object Relations, the Self and the Group. London, Routledge & Kegan Paul.

Bacigalupe, G. (1996) Writing in therapy: a participatory approach, Journal of Family Therapy, 18, p. 389-395.

Bakhtin, M. (1975) The Dialogic Imagination. Austin, TX: University of Texas Press.

Barbules, N.C. (1993) Dialogue in Teaching. New York: Teachers College Press.

Bateson, G. & Ruesch, J. (1951) Communication: The Social Matrix of Psychiatry. New York: W.W. Norton.

Becker, C., Chasin, L., Chasin, R., Herzig, M., & Roth, S. (1995) From stuck debate to new conversation on controversial issues: A report from the Public Conversations Project. Journal of Feminist Family Therapy, 7, (1 and 2), p. 143-163.

Becker, C. et al. (2003) From stuck debates to new conversation on controversial issues: A report from the Public Conversations Project. In M. Gergen and K. Gergen (Eds.) Social Construction, a Reader. London: Sage. p. 182-192.

Beer, C.W. (1910) A Mind that Found Itself. An Autobiography. New York: Longmans, Green.

Bellah, R.N. et al. (1985) Habits of the Heart. Berkeley, CA: University of California Press.

Berg, I.K. & De Shazer, S. (1993) Making numbers talk: Language in therapy. In S. Friedman (Ed.) The New Language of Change: Constructive Collaboration in Psychotherapy. New York: Guilford Press.

Berger, P.L. & Luckmann, T. (1966) The Social Construction of Reality: A Treatise in the Sociology of Knowledge. New York: Doubleday/ Anchor Books.

Berman, M. (1982) All That's Solid Melts into Air: The Experiences of Modernity. New York: Simon and Schuster.

Bertolino, B. & O'Hanlon, W.H. (2001) Collaborative, Competency-based Counseling and Therapy. New York: Allyn and Bacon.

Bierce, A. (1957) The Devil's Dictionary. New York: Sagamore Press.

Billig, M. (1996) Arguing and Thinking. Cambridge: Cambridge University Press, 2nd edition.

Blackman, L. (2001) Hearing Voices: Embodiment and Experience. London: Free Association Books.

Blum, J.D. (1978) On changes in psychiatric diagnosis overtime. American Psychologist, 33, p. 1017-1031.

Bolen, J. (1996) Close to the Bone: Life-threatening Illness and the Search for Meaning. New York: Scribner.

Borgmann, A. (1992) Crossing the Postmodern Divide. Chicago, IL: University of Chicago Press.

Boscolo, L., Cecchin, G., Hoffman, L., & Penn, P. (1988) Familientherapie—Systemtherapie. Das Mailänder Modell. Dortmund: Verlag Modernes Lernen.

Bowker, G.C. & Star, S.L. (1999) Sorting Things Out: Classification and its Consequences. Cambridge, MA: MIT Press.

Boyle, M. (1991) Schizophrenia. A Scientific Delusion. London: Routledge.

Breggin, P.R. (1994) Toxic Psychiatry is Why Therapy, Empathy and Love Must Replace the Drugs, Electroshock, and Biochemical Theories of the "New Psychiatry". New York: St. Martin's Griffin.

_____ (2000) <u>Your Drug May be Your Problem: How and Why to Stop Taking Psychiatric Medication</u>. New York: Perseus.

Breggin & Breggin, G.R. (1995) <u>Talking Back To Prozac: What Doctors Won't Tell You About Today's Most Controversial Drug</u>. New York: St. Martin's.

Brodsky, A.M. & Hare-Mustin, R.T. (1980) <u>Women and Psychotherapy: An Assessment of Research and Practice</u>. New York: Guilford.

Brown, L.S. (1994) <u>Subversive Dialogues: Theory in Feminist Therapy</u>. New York: Basic Books.

_____ (2000) Discomforts of the powerless: Feminist constructions of distress. In R.A. Neimeyer & J.D. Raskin (Eds.) <u>Constructions of Disorder, Meaning-making Frameworks for Psychotherapy</u>. Washington, D.C.: American Psychological Association Press.

Brown, L.S. & Root, M.P.P., (Eds.) (1990) <u>Diversity and Complexity in Feminist Therapy</u>. New York: Haworth.

Bruner, J. (1986) <u>Actual Minds, Possible Worlds</u>. Cambridge, MA: Harvard University Press.

Bruner, J. (1990) <u>Acts of Meaning</u>. Cambridge, MA: Harvard University Press.

Bruner, J. (1996) <u>The Culture of Education</u>. Cambridge, MA: Harvard University Press.

Bugenthal, J.F.T. (1965) <u>The Search for Authenticity</u>. New York: Holt, Rinehart & Winston.

Burkitt, I. (1999) <u>Bodies of Thought</u>. London: Sage.

Butler, M.H., Gardner, B. C., & Bird, M.H. (1998) Not just a time-out: change dynamics of prayer for religious couple in conflict situations. <u>Family Process</u>, 37, p. 451-475.

Califano speaks on health care costs at Grace Square celebration, (1984) Psychiatric News, p. 14.

Caplan, P.J. (1995) They Say You're Crazy: How the World's Most Powerful Psychiatrists Decide Who's Normal. Reading, MA: Addison-Wesley.

Castel, R., Castel, F., & Lovell, A. (1982) The Psychiatric Society. New York: Columbia University Press.

Cecchin, G., Lane, G., & Ray, W.A. (1992) Irreverence: A Strategy for Therapist's Survival. London: Karnac Books.

Chamberlin, J. (1990) The ex-patient's movement: where we've been and where we're going. Journal of Mind and Behavior, II, p. 323-326.

Charlton, J.I. (1998) Nothing About Us Without Us, Disability Oppression and Empowerment. Berkeley: University of California Press.

Cole, M. (1996) Cultural Psychology. Cambridge, MA: Harvard University Press.

Combs, G. & Freedman, J. (1990) Symbol, Story, and Ceremony: Using Metaphor in Individual and Family Therapy. New York: W.W. Norton.

Connor, S. (1989) Postmodernist Culture. Oxford: Blackwell.

Cooperrider, D. & Whitney, D. (2003) Appreciative inquiry. In M. Gergen & K. Gergen (Eds.) Social Construction. A Reader. London: Sage. p. 173-181.

Coyne, J.C. (1982) A brief introduction to epistobabble. Family Therapy Networker, 6(4), p. 27-28.

Cushman, P. (1995) Constructing the Self, Constructing America. A Cultural History of Psychotherapy. Reading, MA: Addison-Wesley.

Cushman, P. & Guilford, P. (2000) Will managed care change our way of being? American Psychologist, 55, p. 985-996.

De Shazer, S. (1994) Words were Originally Magic. New York: W.W. Norton.

Donald, A. (2001) The Wal-Marting of American psychiatry: An ethnography of psychiatric practice in the late 20th Ccentury. Culture, Medicine, and Psychiatry, 25, p. 427-439.

Donley, C. & Budkley, S. (Eds.) (2000) What's Normal? Narratives of Mental and Emotional Disorders. Kent, OH: Kent State University Press.

Drath, W. (2001) The Deep Blue Sea, Rethinking the Source of Leadership. San Francisco, CA: Jossey Bass.

Edelman, M. (1974) The political language of the helping professions. Politics and Society, 4, p. 295-310.

Edwards, D. & Potter, J. (1992) Discursive Psychology. London: Sage.

Efran, J.S. & Clarfield, L.E. (1992) Constructionist therapy, sense and nonsense. In S. McNamee & K. J. Gergen (Eds.), Therapy as Social Construction. Newbury Park, CA: Sage, p. 200-217.

Egelund, M. (1997) (Ed) Enforskel der gor Enforskel: Reflekterende Proceser hos Born, Foroeldre og Personale pa en Doninstitution. Kobenhaven: Hans Reitzels Forlag.

Elkaim, M. (1990) If You Love Me, Don't Love Me: Undoing Reciprocal Double Binds and Other Methods of Change in Couple and Family Therapy. New York: Basic Books.

_____. (Ed.) (1995) Panorama des Therapies Familiales. Paris: Editions Seuil.

Epstein, E.K. (1992) The separation of family- therapeutic theories from social life conditions. PP-Aktuell, 1 and 2, p. 28-41.

Epstein, E.K., Epstein, M.K., & Wiesner, M. (1998) From the reflecting team to the reflexive process: Reflexive cooperation in a psychiatric facility for children and adolescents. In J. Hargens and A. von Schlippe (Eds.) Das Spiel der Ideen. Dortmund: Borgmann, p. 31-52.

Epston, D. & White, M. (1989) Literate Means to Therapeutic Ends. Adelaide: Dulwich Centre Publications.

Epston, D. & White, M. (Eds.) (1992) Experience, Contradiction, Narrative and Imagination. Adelaide, South Australia: Dulwich Centre Publications.

Epston, D., White, M., & Murray, K. (1992) A proposal for a re-authoring therapy: Rose's revisioning of her life and a commentary. In S. McNamee & K.J. Gergen (Eds.) Therapy as Social Construction. Newbury Park, CA: Sage, p. 96-115.

Farber, S. (1990) Institutional mental health & social control: The ravages of epistemological hubris. Journal of Mind and Behavior, 11, p. 285-300.

_____. (1993) Madness, Heresy, and the Rumor of Angels, the Revolt against the Mental Health System. Peru, IL: Open Court.

_____. (1999) Unholy Madness, the Church's Surrender to Psychiatry. Downers Grove, IL: Varsity Press.

Farrelly-Hansen, M. & Bowman, D. (2001) Spirituality and Art Therapy. London: Jessica Kingsley.

Fischer, E. (2000) Linguistic Creativity, Exercises in Philosophical Therapy. Dordrecht: Kluwer.

Fish, S. (1980) Is There a Text in This Class? The Authority of Interpretive Communities. Cambridge: Harvard University Press.

Fishbane, M.D. (2001) Relational narratives of the self. Family Process, 40, p. 273-291.

Flores, M.T. & Carey, G. (2000) Family Therapy with Hispanics: Toward Appreciating Diversity. New York: Allyn and Bacon.

Foucault, M. (1975) Discipline and Punish: The Birth of the Prison. Paris: Gallimard.

_____. (1976) The History of Sexuality Volume 1: An Introduction. Paris: Gallimard.

_____ (1980) Power/Knowledge: Selected Interviews and Other Writings, 1972-1977. New York: Pantheon.

Fowers, B.J. & Richardson, F.C. (1996) Individualism, family ideology and family therapy. Theory and Psychology, 6, p. 121-151.

Fox, D.R. & Prilleltensky, I. (Eds.) (1997) Critical Psychology: An Introduction. London: Sage.

Frascina, F. & Harrison, C. (Eds.) (1982) Modern Art and Modernism. London: Open University Press.

Freedman, J. & Combs, G. (1996) Narrative Therapy: The Social Construction of Preferred Realities. New York: W.W. Norton.

Freeman, J., Epston D., & Lobovits, D. (1997) Playful Approaches to Serious Problems: Narrative therapy with Children and Their Families. New York: W.W. Norton.

Freud, S. (1953) Three essays on the theory of sexuality. In J. Strachey (Ed. and Trans.). The Standard Edition of the Complete Psychological Works of Sigmund Freud. (Vol. 7, pp. 125- 243). London: Hogarth Press. (Original work published 1905).

Friedman, S. (1993) The New Language of Change. New York: Guilford Press.

_____. (Ed.) (1995) The Reflecting Team in Action. New York: Guilford Press.

Frisby, D. (1985) <u>Fragments of Modernity</u>. Cambridge: Polity Press.

Fromm, E. (1976) <u>Escape from Freedom</u>. New York: Avon.

Gadamer, H.G. (1996). <u>Truth and Methods</u>. New York: Seabury. (Originally published in 1960.)

Garfinkel, H. (1967) <u>Studies in Ethnomethodology</u>. Englewood Cliffs, NJ: Prentice-Hall.

Gergen, K.J. (1985) The social constructionist movement in modern psychology. <u>American Psychologist</u>, 40, p. 266-275.

_____ (1992) <u>The polymorphous perversity of the postmodern era</u>. Opening discussion, Family Therapy Networker Conference, Washington D.C., May.

_____ (1993) Foreword. In S. Friedman (Ed.) <u>The New Language of Change: Constructive Collaboration in Psychotherapy</u>. New York: Guilford Press, p. 9-11.

_____ (1994) <u>Realities and Relationships. Soundings in Social Construction</u>. Cambridge, MA: Harvard University Press.

_____ (1994a) <u>Toward Transformation in Social Knowledge</u>. 2nd ed. London: Sage.

_____ (1994b) The limits of pure critique. In H.A. Simons and Michael Billig (Eds.). <u>After Postmodernism: Reconstructing Ideology</u>. Newbury Park, CA: Sage, p. 58-78.

_____ (1996) Technology and the self: from the essential to the sublime. In D. Grodin and T.R. Lidndlof (Eds.) <u>Constructing the Self in a Mediated World: Inquiries in Social Construction</u>. Thousand Oaks, CA, Sage.

_____ (1999) <u>An Invitation to Social Construction</u>. London: Sage.

_____ (2001) <u>Social Construction in Context</u>. London: Sage.

_____ (2001) The Saturated Self. 2nd. ed. New York: Perseus, 2nd edition.

Gergen, K.J. & Davis, K.E. (Eds.) (1985) The Social Construction of the Person. New York: Springer Verlag.

Gergen, K.J. & Gergen, M.M. (1986) Narrative form and the construction of psychological science. In T.R. Sarbin (Ed.) Narrative Psychology: The Storied Nature of Human Conduct. New York: Praeger.

Gergen, K.J. & Gergen, M.M. (1988) Narrative and the self as relationship. In L. Berkowitz (Ed.). Advances in Experimental Social Psychology. New York: Academic Press, vol. 21, p. 17-56.

Gergen, M.M. (2001) Feminist Reconstructions in Psychology: Narrative, Gender, and Performance. Thousand Oaks, CA: Sage.

Gergen, M.M. & Gergen, K.J. (1984) The social construction of narrative accounts. In K.J. Gergen and M.M. Gergen (Eds.) Historical Social Psychology. Hillsdale, NJ: Erlbaum, p. 173-189.

Gergen, M.M. & Gergen, K.J. (1993) Narratives of the gendered body in popular autobiography. In R. Josselson and A. Lieblich (Eds.) The Narrative Study of Lives. Newbury Park, CA: Sage, p. 191-218.

Gilligan, C. (1982) In a Different Voice. Cambridge, MA: Harvard University Press.

Gilligan, S.G. (1996) The relational self: the expanding of love beyond desire. In M.F. Hoyt (Ed.) Constructive Therapies, Volume 2. New York: Guilford Press, p. 211-237.

Glaserfeld, E. von (1988) The reluctance to change a way of thinking. Irish Journal of Psychology, 9, p. 82-90.

Glass, J.M. (1993) Shattered Selves: Multiple Personality in a Postmodern World. Ithaca, NY: Cornell University Press.

Goffman, E. (1961) Asylums: Essays on the Social Situation of Mental Patients and Other Inmates. Garden City, NJ: Doubleday.

Goncalves, O.F. (1995) Cognitive narrative psychotherapy: the hermeneutic construction of alternative meanings. In M.J. Mahoney (Ed.) Cognitive and Constructive Psychotherapies. New York: Springer.

Goolishian, H. & Anderson, H. (1987) Language systems and therapy: an evolving idea. Psychotherapy, 24, (3S), p. 529-538.

Gordon, C. & Gergen, K.J. (Eds.) (1968) The Self in Social Interaction. New York: Wiley.

Gordon, R.A. (1990) Anorexia and Bulimia. Cambridge: Basil Blackwell.

Graumann, C.F. & Gergen, K.J. (Eds.) (1993) Historical Dimensions of Psychological Discourse. New York: Cambridge University Press.

Griffith, J.L. & Griffith, M.E. (1992) Therapeutic change in religious families. Working with the God-construct. In L.A Burton (Ed.) Religion and the Family. Binghampton, NY: Haworth Press.

_____ (2001) Encountering the Sacred in Psychotherapy. New York: Guilford.

Gross, M.L. (1978) The Psychological Society. New York: Random House.

Grove, D.R. (1993) Ericksonian therapy with multiple personality clients. Journal of Family Psychotherapy. Vol. 4, 2nd edition, p. 136.

Habermas, J. (1975) Legitimation Crisis. Boston: Beacon Press.

Hacking, I. (1995) Rewriting the soul: Multiple Personality and the Science of Memory. Princeton: Princeton University Press.

Hare-Mustin, R., & Marecek, J., (1988) The meaning of difference. Gender theory, postmodernism, and psychology. American Psychologist, 43, p. 455-464.

262   Therapeutic Realities

Hartmann, H. (1960) Psychoanalysis and Moral Values. New York: International Universities Press.

Harvey, D. (1989) The Condition of Postmodernity. Oxford: Blackwell.

Harwood, H.J., Napolitano, D.M., & Kristiansen, P.L. (1983) Economic Costs to Society of Alcohol and Drug Abuse and Mental Illness. Research Triangle, NC: Research Triangle Institute.

Heinrichs, R.W. (2001) In Search of Madness: Schizophrenia and Neuroscience. New York: Oxford University Press.

Held, B.S. (1996) Back to Reality. a Critique of Postmodern Psychotherapy. New York: Norton.

Hepworth, J. (1999) The Social Construction of Anorexia Nervosa. London: Sage.

Hermans, C.A.M., Immink, G., de Jong, A., & van der Lans, J. (Eds.) (2001) Social Constructionism and Theology. Leyde: Brill.

Hermanns, H.J.M. & Kempen, H.J.G. (1993) The Dialogical Self: Meaning as Movement. San Diego: Academic Press.

Hermanns, H.J.M., Kempen,H.J.G., & Van Loon, R.J.P. (1992) The dialogical self: beyond individualism and rationalism. American Psychologist, 47, p. 23-33.

Hillman, J. & Ventura, M. (1992) We've Had a Hundred Years of Psychotherapy and the World's Getting Worse. New York: HarperCollins.

Hoffman, L. (1990) Constructing realities: an art of lenses. Family Process, 29, p. 1-12.

Hoffman, L. (1993) Exchanging Voices: A Collaborative Approach to Family Therapy. London: Karnac Books.

_____ (2002) Family Therapy: An Intimate History. New York: Norton.

Horney, K. (1950) Neurosis and Human Growth. New York: Norton.

Holzman, L. & Mendez, R. (Eds.) (2003) Psychological Investigations, a Clinician's Guide to Social Therapy. New York: Brunner-Rutledge.

Hoyt, M.F. (1994a) Constructive Therapies. New York: Guilford Press.

_____ (1994b) On the importance of keeping it simple and taking the patient seriously: a conversation with Steve de Shazer and John Weakland. In M.F. Hoyt (Ed.) Constructive Therapies. New York: Guilford Press, p. 11-40.

_____ (Ed.) (1996) Constructive Therapies, Volume 2. New York: Guilford Press.

_____ (1998) The Handbook of Constructive Therapies. San Francisco, CA: Jossey-Bass.

_____ (2000) Some Stories Are Better than Others. New York: Brunner-Mazel.

_____ (2001) Interviews with Brief Therapy Experts. Philadelphia, PA: Brunner-Routledge.

Hoyt, M.F. & Ordover, J. (1988) Book review of J.F. Zeig (Ed.) The Evolution of Psychotherapy. In Imagination, Cognition, and Personality. Vol. 8, 2nd edition, p. 181-186.

Hustvedt, S. (2003) What I Loved. London: Hodder and Stoughton.

Hutschemaekers, G. (1989) Neurosen in Nederland. Nijmegen: Sun.

Ibanez, T.G. (1992) Como se puede no ser constructivista hoy en dia? Revista de Psicoterapia. Vol. 3, 12th edition, p. 17-27.

Ingleby, D. (1980) Understanding mental illness. In D. Ingleby (Ed.) Critical Psychiatry: The Politics of Mental Health. New York: Pantheon, p. 23-71.

Jennings, S. & Minde, A. (1994) Art Therapy and Dramatherapy. London: Jessica Kingsley.

Jordan, J.V., Kaplan, A.G., Miller, J.B. Stiver, I.P., & Surrey, J.L. (Eds.) (1991) Women's Growth in Connection: Writings from the Stone Center. New York: Guilford.

Kabat Zinn, J. (2005) Coming to Our Senses. New York: Hyperion.

Karrass, C.L. (1992) The Negotiating Game. New York: HarperCollins.

Kegan, R. (1994) In Over Our Heads: The Mental Demands of Modern Life. Cambridge, MA: Harvard University Press.

Kelly, G.A. (1955) A Theory of Personality: The Psychology of Personal Constructs. 2 Vol., New York: Norton.

Kiesler, C.A. & Sibulkin, A.E. (1987) Mental Hospitalization: Myths and Facts about a National Crisis. Newbury Park, CA: Sage.

Kirk, S.A. & Kutchins, H. (1992) The Selling of DSM: The Rhetoric of Science in Psychiatry. Hawthorne, NY: Aldine de Gruyter.

Kogan, S.M. & Brown, A.C. (1998) Reading against the lines: resisting foreclosure in therapy discourse. Family Process, 37, p. 495-512.

Kovel, J. (1980) The American mental health industry. In D. Ingleby (Ed.) Critical Psychiatry: The Politics of Mental Health. New York: Pantheon, p. 72-101.

_____ (1988) The Radical Spirit: Essays on Psychoanalysis and Society. London: Free Press.

Kramer, P.D. (2005) Against Depression. New York: Viking.

Kuhn, T.S. (1970) The Structure of Scientific Revolutions. Chicago, IL: University of Chicago Press.

Kukla, R., Veroff, J., & Douvan, E. (1979) Social class and the use of professional help for personal problems: 1957-1976. Journal of Health and Social Behavior, 26, p. 2-17.

Kutchins, H. & Kirk, S.A. (1997) Making Us Crazy, DSM: The Psychiatric Bible and the Creation of Mental Disorders. New York: Free Press.

Laing, R.D. (1967) The Politics of Experience. Harmondsworth/New York: Penguine/Ballantine Books.

Lange, A. (1996) Using writing assignments with families managing legacies of extreme traumas. Journal of Family Therapy, 18, p. 375-388.

Lane, R.D., Nadel, L., & Ahern, G. (Ed.) (1999) Cognitive Neuroscience of Emotion. New York: Oxford University Press.

Lannamann, J.W. (1998) Social construction and materiality: The limits of indeterminacy in therapeutic settings. Family Process, 47, p. 393-413.

Lasch, C. (1979) The Culture of Narcissism. New York: Norton.

Latour, B. (1987) Science in Action. Cambridge, MA: Harvard University Press.

Lax, W.D. (1992) Postmodern thinking in a clinical practice. In S. McNamee & K. Gergen (Eds.) Therapy as Social Construction. London: Sage, p. 69-85.

Lehmann, P. (Ed.) (2004) Coming off Psychiatric Drugs. Berlin: Peter Lehmann.

_____ (2005) All about PSY DREAM, Psychiatric drug registration, evaluation and all-inclusive monitoring. Epidemiologia e Psichiatra Sociale, 14, p. 15-21.

Leifer, R. (1990) The medical model as the ideology of the therapeutic state. Journal of Mind and Behavior, 11, p. 247-258.

Lerman, H. (1996) Pigeonholing Women's Misery: A History and Critical Analysis of the Psychodiagnosis of Women in the Twentieth Century. New York: Basic Books.

Levin, S., London, S., & Tarragona, M. (Eds.) (1998) Hearing more voices: Beyond traditions in writing, research, and therapy. Journal of Systemic Therapies, 17 (4).

Levin, F.M. (2003) Mapping the Mind: The Intersection of Psychoanalysis and Neuroscience. New York: Karnac.

Lifton, R. (1987) The Future of Immortality. New York: Basic Books.

London, P. (1986) The Modes and Morals of Psychotherapy. (2nd edition). New York: Hemisphere.

Lutz, C. A. (1998) Unnatural Emotions: Everyday Sentiments on a Micronesian Atoll and their Challenge to Western Theory. Chicago, IL: University of Chicago Press.

Lyotard, J.F. (1984) The Postmodern Condition. Paris: De Minuit.

MacKinnon, L.K. & Miller, D. (1987) The new epistemology and the Milan approach: feminist and sociopolitical considerations. Journal of Marital and Family Therapy, 13, p. 139-155.

Madogam, S. & Epston, D. (1995) From "spy-chiatric" gaze to communities of concern: from professional monologue to dialogue. In S. Friedman (Ed.) The Reflecting Team in Action. New York: Guilford Press.

Mahler, M.S., Bergman, A., & Pine, F. (1975) The Psychological Birth of the Human Infant. New York: Basic Books.

Mahoney, M.J. (Ed.) (1995) The Cognitive and Constructive Psychotherapies. New York: Springer Verlag.

Malchiodi, C.A. (2000) Art Therapy and Computer Technology. London: Jessica Kingsley.

Mancuso, J.C. (1996) Constructionism, personal construct psychology and narrative psychology. Theory and Psychology, 6, p. 47-70.

Margolis, J. (1966) Psychotherapy and Morality. New York: Random House.

Martin, E. (2000) The rationality of mania. In R. Reid & S. Traweek (Eds.) Doing Science and Culture. London: Rutledge.

Martin, E. (2004) Talking back to neuro-reductionism. In H. Thomas & J. Ahmcd (Eds.) Cultural Bodies: Ethnography and Theory. Oxford: Blackwell.

Martin, J. & Sugarman, J. (1999) The Psychology of Human Possibility and Constraint. Albany, NY: State University of New York Press.

Masserman, J.H. (1960) Psychoanalysis and Human Values. New York: Grune & Stratton.

Masson, J.M. (1994) Against Therapy. Monroe, ME: Common Courage Press.

Maturana, H.R. & Varela, F. J. (1987) The Tree of Knowledge. Boston, MA: New Science Library.

McAdams, D.P. (1993) The Stories We Live By. New York: William Morrow.

McLeod, J. (1997) Narrative and Psychotherapy. London: Sage.

_____ J. (Ed.) (2003) Handbook of Narrative and Psychotherapy. London: Sage.

McLuhan, M. (1964) Understanding Media: The Extension of Man. New York: Signet.

McNamee, S. & Gergen, K.J. (Eds.) (1992) Therapy as Social Construction. London: Sage.

McNamee, S. & Gergen, K.J. (1999) Relational Responsibility. Thousand Oaks, CA: Sage.

Mead, G.H. (1934) Mind, Self and Society. Chicago, IL: University of Chicago Press.

Mechanic, D. (1980) Mental Health and Social Policy. Englewood Cliffs, NJ: Prentice-Hall.

Metzl, J.M. (2003) Prozac on the Couch, Prescribing Gender in the Era of Wonder Drugs. Durham: Duke University Press.

Middleton, D. & Edwards, D. (Eds.) (1990) Collective Remembering. London: Sage.

Mitchell, S.A. (1993) Hope and Dread in Psychoanalysis. New York: Basic Books.

Mitchell, S. (2000) Relationality. From Object Relations to Intersubjectivity. New York: Analytic Press.

Morrison, M. (1994) The evolution of Tom Hanks. Us, The Entertainment Magazine, August, p. 46-52.

Murphy, M. (1997) Relationship-centeredness, the essential nature of human health care. Human Health Care, 13, p. 142-143.

Neimeyer, R.A. (1999) Narrative strategies in grief therapy. Journal of Constructivist Psychology, 12, p. 65-86.

_____ (Ed.) (2001) Meaning Reconstruction and the Experience of Loss. Washington, D.C.: American Psychological Association.

Neimeyer, R.A. & Freixas, G. (1990) Constructivist contributions to psychotherapy integration. Journal of Integrative and Eclectic Psychotherapy, 9, p. 4-20.

Neimeyer, R.A. & Mahoney, M.J. (Eds.) (1995) Constructivism in Psychotherapy. Washington, D.C.: American Psychological Association.

Neimeyer, R.A. & Raskin, J.D. (Eds.) (2000) Constructions of Disorder: Meaning-Making Frameworks for Psychotherapy. Washington, D.C.: American Psychological Association.

Newham, P. (1999) Using Voice and Movement in Therapy. London: Jessica Kingsley.

Newman, F. (1991) The Myth of Psychology. New York: Castillo.

Newman, F. & Holzman, L. (1996) Unscientific Psychology: A Cultural Performatory Approach to Understanding Human Life. Westport, CT: Praeger.

Newman, F. & Holzman, L. (1999) Beyond narrative to performed conversation. Journal of Constructivist Psychology, 12, p. 23-41.

O'Hanlon, W.H. (1993) Possibility therapy: from iatrogenic injury to iatrogenic healing. In S. Gilligan & R. Price (Eds.) Therapeutic Conversations. New York: W.W. Norton.

_____ (1994) Thriving through Crisis: Turn Tragedy and Trauma into Growth and Change. New York: Perigree.

_____ (1999) Evolving Possibilities: Selected Works of Bill O'Hanlon. New York: Brunner-Routledge.

O'Hanlon, B. & Rowan, T. (1999) Solution-Oriented Therapy for Chronic and Severe Mental Illness. New York: Norton.

O'Hanlon, W.H. & Weiner-Davis, M. (1989) In Search of Solutions: A New Direction in Psychotherapy. New York: W.W. Norton.

Paglia, C (1992) Junk bonds and corporate raiders: Academe in the hour of the wolf. In C. Paglia Sex, Art, and American Culture: Essays. New York: Vintage, p. 170-248.

Pakman, M. (2000) Disciplinary knowledge, postmodernism and globalization: A call for critical social practices in human services. Cybernetics and Human Knowing, 7, p. 105-126.

Parker, I. (1998) Against postmodernism: psychology in cultural context. Theory and Psychology, 9, p. 601-627.

_____ (1998) (Ed.) Social Constructionism, Discourse, and Realism. London: Sage.

Paré, D.A. (2002) Discursive Wisdom: Reflections on Ethics and Therapeutic Knowledge. International Journal of Critical Psychology, 7, p. 30-52.

Paré, D.A. & Larner, G. (eds.) (2004) Collaborative Practice in Psychology and Therapy. Binghamton, NY: Haworth Press.

Parry, A. & Doan, R.E. (1994) Story Re-visions: Narrative Therapy in the Postmodern World. New York: Guilford Press.

Peeters, H. (1995) The historical vicissitudes of mental diseases, their character and treatment. In C. Graumann & K. Gergen (Eds.) The Historical Context of Psychological Discourse. London: Sage.

Penn, P. (1982) Circular questioning. Family Process, Vol. 21, p. 267-280.

_____ (1985) Feed-forward: future questions, future maps. Family Process, Vol. 24, p. 299-310.

_____ (2001) Chronic illness. Trauma, language and writing. Family Process, 40, 1, p. 33-52.

Penn, P. & Frankfurt, M. (1994) Creating a participant text: writing, multiple voices, narrative multiplicity. Family Process, 33, p. 217-231.

Penn, P. & Frankfurt, M. (1999) A circle of voices. In S. McNamee & K. Gergen, Relational Responsibility. London: Sage.

Polkinghorne, D.E. (1988) Narrative Knowing in the Human Sciences. Albany, NY: State University Press of New York.

Raelin, J.A. (2003) Creating Leaderful Organizations. San Francisco, CA: Berett-Koehler.

Reason, P. & Bradbury, H. (Eds.) (2001) Handbook of Action Research. London: Sage.

Restak, R. (2003) The New Brain: How the Modern Age is Rewiring Your Mind. New York: Rodale.

Richard, P.S. & Bergin, A.E. (1997) A Spiritual Strategy for Counseling and Psychotherapy. Washington, D.C.: American Psychological Association.

Ricoeur, P. (1979) The model of the text: meaningful action considered as a text. In P. Rabinow & W. Sullivan (Eds.) Interpretive Social Science: A Reader. Berkeley: University of California Press.

Riikonen, E. & Smith, G.M. (1997) Re-Imagining Therapy: Living Conversation and Relational Knowing. London: Sage.

Rogers, C. (1951) Client-Centered Therapy: Its Current Practice, Implications and Theory. London: Constable.

Rose, N.S. (1985) The Psychological Complex. London: Routledge & Kegan Paul.

Rosen, G. (1968) Madness in Society. Chicago, IL: Chicago University Press.

Rosen, H. & Kuehlwein K.T. (Eds.) (1996) Constructing Realities: Meaning-Making Perspectives for Psychotherapists. San Francisco, CA: Jossey-Bass.

Rosenbaum, R. & Dyckman, J. (1996) No self? No problem! Actualizing empty sell in psychotherapy. In M. F. Hoyt (Ed.) Constructive Therapies, Volume 2. New York: Guilford Press, p. 238-274.

Ryder, R.G. (1987) The Realistic Therapist: Modesty and Relativism in Therapy and Research. New Park, CA: Sage.

Sadler, J.Z. (Ed.) (2002) Descriptions and Prescriptions, Values, Mental Disorder, and the DSMs. Baltimore: Johns Hopkins University Press.

Sarbin, T.R. (Ed.) (1986) Narrative Psychology: The Storied Nature of Human Conduct. New York: Praeger.

Sarbin, T.R. & Mancuso, J.C. (1980) Schizophrenia: Medical Diagnosis or Verdict? Elsmford, New York: Pergamon.

Sass, L.A. (1992) Madness and Modernism: Insanity in the Light of Modern Art, Literature, and Thought. New York: Basic Books.

Schacht, T.E. (1985) DSM—III and the politics of truth. American Psychologist, 40, p. 513-521.

Schafer, R. (1992) Retelling a Life: Narration and Dialogue in Psychoanalysis. New York: Basic Books.

Schnitman, D.F. (1996) Between the extant and the possible. Journal of Constructivist Psychology, 9, p. 263-282.

Schwartz, J.M. & Begley, S. (2002) The Mind and the Brain: Neuroplasticity and the Power of Mental Force. New York: Regan.

Schwarz, R.A. (1998) From "either-or" to "both-and": treating dissociative disorders collaboratively. In M.F. Hoyt (Ed.) The Handbook of Constructive Therapies. San Francisco, CA: Jossey-Bass, p. 428-448.

Segal, Z.V., Williams, M.G, & Teasdale, J.D. (2002) Mindfulness Based Cognitive Therapy for Depression, A New Approach. New York: Guilford.

Seikkula, J. (1995) Psychosis—A voice about the current dialogue. Zeitschrift für systemische Therapie, 13, 3, p. 183-192.

_____ (1996) Combining family and hospital. In T. Keller and N. Greve (Eds.) Systemische Praxis in der Psychiatrie. Bonn: Psychiatrie-Verlag, p. 303-321.

Seikkula, J. et al. (1995) Treating psychosis by means of open dialogue. In S. Friedman (Ed.) The Reflective Process in Action. New York: Guilford.

Selvini-Palazzoli, M, Boscolo, L., Cecchin, G., & Prata, G. (1980) Hypothesizing, circularity, neutrality: three guidelines for the conduct of the session. Family Process, 19, p. 3-12.

Semin, G.R. & Gergen, K.J. (Eds.) (1990) Everyday Understanding: Social and Scientific Implications. Newbury Park, CA: Sage.

Sheff, T.J. (1966) Being Mentally Ill: A Sociological Theory. Chicago, IL: Aldine.

Sheinberg, M. & Penn, P. (1991) Gender dilemmas, gender questions and the gender mantra. Journal of Marital and Family Therapy, 17, p. 33-44.

Shotter, J. (1984) Social Accountability and Selfhood. Oxford: Blackwell.

_____ (1993) Conversational Realities. London: Sage.

Sinaikin, P. (2004) Coping with the medical model in clinical practice or "How I learned to stop worrying and love DSM" Journal of Critical Psychology, Counselling and Psychotherapy. 4, p. 36-48.

Sluzki, C.E. (1992) Transformations: a blueprint for narrative changes in therapy. Family Process, 31, p. 217-230.

Snyder, M. (1996) Our "other history": poetry as a metaphor for narrative therapy. Journal of Family Therapy, 18, p. 337-359.

Solomon, A. (2001) The Noonday Demon, an Atlas of Depression. New York: Touchstone.

Spence, D. (1982) Narrative Truth and Historical Truth: Meaning and Interpretation in Psychoanalysis. New York: Norton.

Spinelli, E. (1994) Demystifying Therapy. London: Constable.

Spitzer, R.L. & Williams, J.B. (1985) Classification of mental disorders. In H.I.Kaplan and B.J. Sadock (Eds.) Comprehensive Textbook of Psychiatry. Baltimore, OH: Williams & Wilkins, p. 580-602.

Steffe, L.P. & Gale, J. (Eds.) (1995) Alternative Epistemologies in Education. Hillsdale, NJ: Erlbaum.

Stein, D.J. (2002) Cognitive-Affective Neuroscience of Depression and Anxiety Disorders. New York: Taylor and Francis.

Suryani, L.K. & Jensen, G.D. (1993) The Balinese People: A Reinvestigation of Character. New York: Oxford University Press.

Susko, M.A. (1991) Cry of the Invisible. Baltimore, OH: Conservatory Press.

Szasz, T.S. (1961) The Myth of Mental Illness: Foundations of a Theory of Personal Conduct. New York: Hoeber-Harper.

_____. (1963) Law, Liberty and Psychiatry: An Inquiry into the Social Uses of Mental Health Practices. New York: Macmillan.

_____ (1970) The Manufacture of Madness: A Comparative Study of the Inquisition and the Mental Health Movement. New York: Harper & Row.

Taggart, M. (1985) The feminist critique in epistemological perspective: questions of context in family therapy. Journal of Marital and Family Therapy, 11, p. 113-126.

Tomm, K. (2001) Honoring our internalized others and the ethics of caring: A conversation with Karl Tomm. In M. F. Hoyt (Ed.) Interviews with Brief Therapy Experts. Philadelphia, PA: Brunner-Routledge.

Turkington, C. (1985) Support helps schizophrenics meet needs. American Psychological Association Monitor, October, p. 5.

Vygotsky, L.S. (1978) Mind in Society: The Development of Higher Psychological Processes. Cambridge, MA: Harvard University Press.

Walsh, F. (Ed.) (1999) Spiritual Resources in Family Therapy. New York: Guilford.

Watzlawick, P. (Ed.) (1984) The Invented Reality. New York: Norton.

Watzlawick, P., Beavin, J.H., and Jackson, D.D. (1967) Pragmatics of Human Communication. New York: Norton.

Weingarten, K. (2003) Common Shock: Witnessing Violence Every Day. New York: Dutton.

Weingarten, K. (1998) The small and the ordinary in the daily practice of a postmodern narrative therapy. Family Process, 37, p. 3-15.

Wertsch, J.V. (1985) Vygotsky and the Social Formation of Mind. Cambridge, MA: Harvard University Press.

Wertsch, J.V. (1991) Voices of the Mind. Cambridge: Cambridge University Press.

West, J.D., Bubenzer, D.L., & Bitter, J.R. (Eds.) (1998) Social Construction in Couple and Family Counseling. Washington, D.C.: American Counseling Association Press.

White, M. & Epston, D. (1990) Narrative Means to Therapeutic Ends. New York: W.W. Norton.

Whorf, B.L. (1956) Language, Thought and Reality. Cambridge: MIT Press.

Wiener, M. (1991) Schizophrenia: a defective, deficient, disrupted, disorganized Concept. In W.F. Flack, Jr., D.R. Miller, & M. Wiener (Eds.) What is Schizophrenia? New York: Springer Verlag.

Wittgenstein, L. (1953) Philosophical Investigations. Trans. G. Anscombe. New York: Macmillan.

Zimmermann, J.L. & Dickerson, V.C. (1996) If Problems Talked: Narrative Therapy in Action. New York: Guilford Press.

Endnotes

1. See, for example, Gergen (1994, 1999, 2001),

2. See, for example, Bellah et al (1985); and Lasch (1979).

3. See, especially Mitchell (1993). For related work in a feminist frame see Jordan et al (1991).

4. See especially Fishbane (2001).

5. See for example, Wertsch's 1985 account.

6. See, for example, Bruner (1990), and Cole (1996).

7. See, for example, Middleton and Edwards (1990) Billig...memory....

8. See Reason and Bradbury(2001).

9. See, for example, Bruner (1996), Barbules (1993).

10. See, for example, Drath (2001), Raelin (2003).

11. See, for example, Cooperrider and Whitney (2003).

12. See, for example, Becker et al. (2003).

13. See for example, Held (1996), Parker (1998).

14. See, for example, Garfinkel (1967), Kuhn (1970), Latour (1987), Edwards and Potter (1994), Fish (1980), and Shotter (1993).

15. You may object: "well, even if not acknowledged, what I say might mean something to me personally," and that may be. But the question then becomes, how did your utterances come to have personal meaning? We take up this issue shortly.

16. A question frequently asked is "what is the essential difference between social constructionism and constructivism?" A definitive answer cannot be offered, because these terms are used in many different contexts and with different and sometimes interchangeable meanings. There is no central ministry

of language to police the meaning. However, there is a central difference that may runs throughout many of these discussions, and is useful to articulate. For many scholars and practitioners, constructivism has its roots in individualist psychology, with Piaget and Kelly serving as early progenitors. From this standpoint it is the individual who constructs the world, and the site of construction is the individual mind. Radical constructivism of the kind elaborated by Ernst von Glasersfeld (1996), represents the logical extension of this view. In contrast, contemporary social constructionism is largely concerned with the construction of the world in language. Thus, the primary site of construction is not within, but *among* people. In this sense, scholars such as Wittgenstein, Bakhtin, Derrida, Latour and Foucault become relevant. This form of constructionism is represented in the present volume. At the same time, the distinction between constructivism and constructionism can be blurred in many ways. Early social construction of the kind espoused by Berger and Luckmann (1966) attempted to integrate both phenomenology (inside the mind) and macro-sociology (external reality). Many traditional constructivists are now sensitive to the constructionist lines of reasoning, and view language as the source of thought, or mental construction (See for example, issues of the Journal of Constructivist Psychology). In similar fashion, many constructionists—including myself—now draw from Vygotsky in reconceptualizing thought as the internal use of language. Convergence is everywhere in motion.

17. See also Hoffman's (2002) extension and elaboration of these ideas in her history of family therapy.

18. For additional discussions of modernism see Berman, 1982; Frisby (1985), Frascina and Harrison (1982), and Gergen (1991).

19. For an extensive account of the problems the modernist (or empiricist foundationalist) orientation to psychotherapy see Ryder(1987).

20. For discussion of the particular relationship between postmodernism and therapeutic practice see Gergen (1991; 1994), Ibanez (1992), and Lax (1992).

21. The chief emphasis of this chapter is on change and flexibility in narrative construction. However, this is in no way to make a principled argument for these ends. Change is stressed primarily because those seeking therapy are typically discontent with the status quo. For those whose world is under threat, stabilizing narratives may be indicated.

22. See Mary Boyle's (1991) careful critique of diagnoses of schizophrenia. As she shows, such diagnoses are not evidentially based, but are highly interpretive, and rife with conceptual confusion. See also Wiener's (1991) critique of the concept of schizophrenia.

23. Also compelling is Murray Edelman's (1974) discussion of the "professional imperialism" of the helping professions. For a more baldly stated case against psychiatry's appropriation of power in the present century see Gross(1978). For additional contributions to a critical understanding of the ways in which mental discourse is employed, see Fox and Prilleltensky (1997), Ingelby (1980), and Breggin (1991).

24. For an extended account of the expansion of psychiatry in the U.S. and the accompanying "psychiatrization of difference" see Castel, Castel, and Lovell (1982).

25. See also Bowker and Star's (1999) volume, <u>Sorting things out, Classification and its consequences</u>. Cambridge: MIT Press.

26. See also Gordon's (1991) analysis of the function of the media in the generation of what we index as anorexia and bulimia.

27. See also Kovel (1988) on psychiatry as a market economy.

28. A case in point is the increase in the use of psychiatric drugs in treating children and teenagers. In less than a ten year period in the US, the use of psychotropic drugs tripled, and with scant research on their efficacy or side-effects (<u>Philadelphia Inquirer</u>, Jan. 14, 2003).

29. For an expansion of this point, see Farber (1999).

30. In his "best seller" volume depicting his personal experience with depression, Andrew Solomon (2001) makes a strong case for the contribution of anti-depressants to his own well-being. The question is not whether drugs should be prescribed in individual cases, but the move toward prescribing them in virtually all cases.

31. See, for example, www.antipsychiatry.org, http://www.adhdfraud.com/, http://www.narpa.org/index.html, http://www.power2u.org/index.html, http://www.stopshrinks.org/, and http://thechp.syr.edu/chp.htm.

32. See, for example, http://www.peoplewho.org/, http://www.hearing-voices.org/ and http://www.webcom.com/thrive/schizo/welcome.shtml.